Pocket Guide for
Zero Point Energy Wanding

The World's #1 ZPE Wanding Guide

Bruce Goldwell & Jean Perrins

Hardcopy ISBN-13: 978-1461136033

Hardcopy ISBN-10: 1461136032

Book Web Site: www.BruceGoldwell.com

Forward

Pain is one of the scourges of modern society. Our lifestyles, diets, workloads and habits demand more of us than we are designed to tolerate. Most of it we do to ourselves. Somehow we lose our way.

This pocket guide is designed to empower you to help your body to heal and for you to help your loved ones as well. One small step at a time is all it takes to bring a renewed glimmer of hope to those trapped in the strangling net of illness, disease and pain.

Remember always that your body has a wonderful capacity to heal itself. It just needs the right conditions and the right opportunities.

The power is in your hands and with a good quality zero-point energy wand in your hands, you now have a direction. Just point the wand, use your intention to feel better and use the enclosed wanding techniques to your heart's content.

We wish you well, always.

Wanding

Techniques

Clockwise Circular Motion

Simply rotate your wanding hand in a clockwise direction. Hold wand tip about one inch from the skin. Three to four rotations per second is a good frequency for most people. In older people you may want to go slower at 1-2 rotations per second as their energy is usually weaker. Older people may respond more slowly as their bodies are more toxic. If you are carrying around a lot of excess cargo, you may also want to wand more slowly. Since this is a more soothing technique and can be a follow-up technique to the cross hatching technique, 5 to 20 minutes is a good time duration for this, depending on whether it is used as the main technique or not.

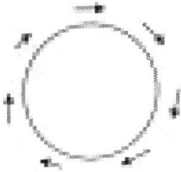

Clockwise Circular Motion with a Dot

This technique is identical to the one above except after each rotation you pretend you are dotting an 'I'. This tends to be more efficient at breaking up congestion and swelling than the circular technique.

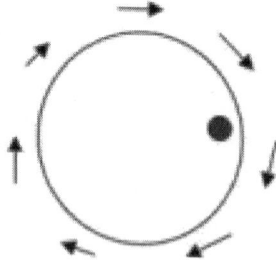

Dotting

This is an up and down technique, vertical to the skin that move the wand about an inch up and down. It is good for swelling and conditions like sinus problems and stuffy noses. About two 'dots' per second is a good rhythm. Ten to fifteen minutes is a good time to do this technique.

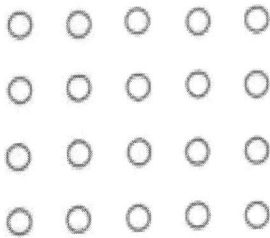

O O O O O

O O O O O

O O O O O

O O O O O

Circle Dipping

A combination of circling and dipping usually with 3-4 circles followed by 1-2 dips. This is very effective for headaches and joint pain. Deeper pain seems to like this method. Since deep pain is harder to get at, you may need to do this technique for about 20 minutes or so to see relief.

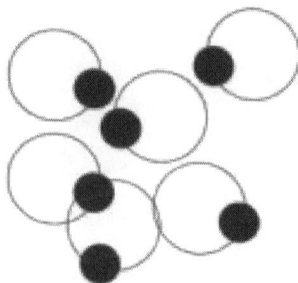

Dipping

This is an in-out motion of about 3 inches with the wand tip coming close to the skin surface. It creates an energy wave penetrating deep into the body. Dipping works well for deep pain and has a rejuvenating effect on tissues. If you have long standing deep pain, this may be the first technique you need to use after the cross hatching technique for approximately 10 minutes.

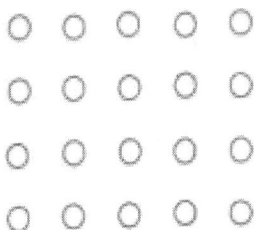

Directional Dipping

This is a swooping motion in the direction of energy flow. Usually this will be used to help drain swelling toward the heart. It is also good for congestion. Ten minutes seems to be a good time for this technique.

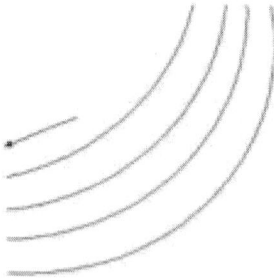

Rolling

This is an awesome technique for working on the soles of the feet. Hold the wand vertically on the skin and roll the wand between your fingers on particular acupressure points on the feet. Use slight to medium pressure on the spot depending how sensitive it is. This is good for deep organ difficulties that the wand cannot reach through other wanding techniques. Ten to 20 minutes is a good time for this technique.

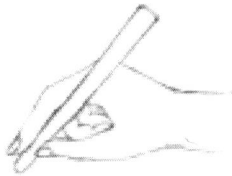

Rubbing

This is another awesome technique for working on the soles of the feet. Hold the wand vertically on the skin and rub the wand back and forth in half inch strokes using slight to medium pressure. This is also good for deep tissue work for organ difficulties. Ten to 20 minutes is a good time for this technique.

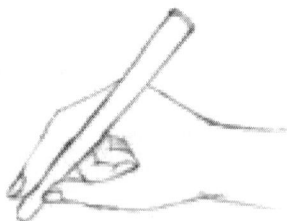

Tip Tapping

Gently tapping the area with the wand tip will frequently get things happening with people who are energy toxic from working in office buildings or using cell phones etc. Having them drink a glass of wanded water frequently helps speed things up as their internal water molecules listen more effectively to the wand energy.

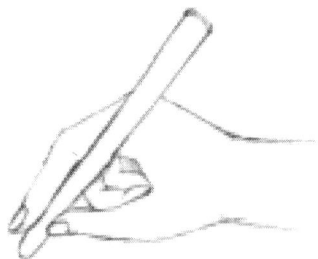

Side Brushing

Using the side of the wand to gently brush the skin is excellent for rashes and bruising as well as for strengthening and rejuvenating the skin tissues. This is an awesome technique for around and under the eyes. You can do it in the evenings while you are watching TV. Since this is a more cosmetic technique, there is no set time for it.

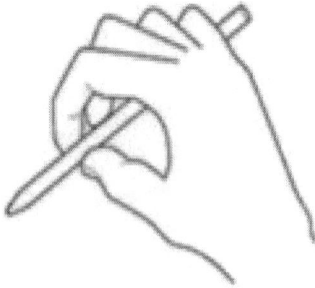

Side Rolling

Rolling the side of the wand over areas of the face that appear to show the signs of aging can help rejuvenate and oxygenate the skin, reducing fine lines and wrinkles. This technique stimulates the production of elastin and collagen in the skin, thus reducing fine lines and wrinkles. There is no set time for this technique either.

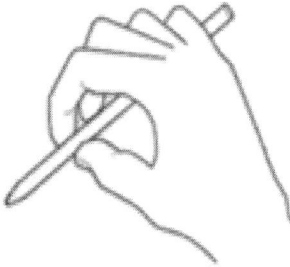

Stroking

Rest the wand on the skin and pull it in long strokes in the direction of the heart. This helps move the stuck energy and gets the innate energy flow going. This is a calming and soothing technique that can be done for any length of time.

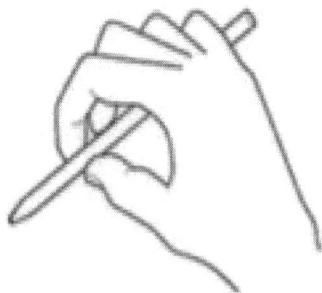

Cross-Hatching

This is a simple back and forth motion with alternating directions. Vertically for ten seconds followed by horizontally for ten seconds and so forth parallel to the skin, is how this technique is done. This action tends to loosen up swelling and allow for drainage of toxins. Always follow with circling to finish! You may need to wand with this technique up to 20 minutes to begin to experience relief.

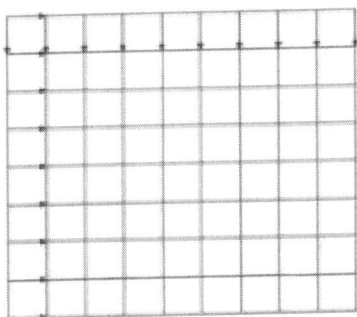

Zigzag Cross Hatching

This technique is like the technique above except you zigzag across the area in both directions, vertically and horizontally.

It breaks up swelling and helps break up lymph congestion under the armpits, in the neck and the sides of the lower abdomen. You may need to use this technique before using a directional dipping technique and do it for a similar time as above.

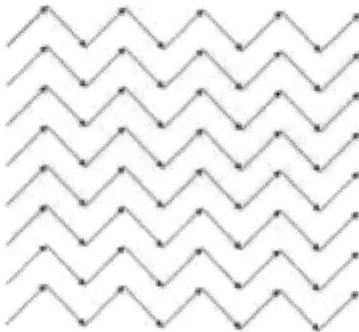

Facelifting

One of the most exciting techniques or combination of techniques is used for refining the skin on the face. This technique called feathering is using vary light, short upward strokes on the neck, chin, and under the lower lip. Diagonal upward feathering strokes are used on the cheeks, upper lip, under the eyes and on the forehead. Around the eyes, gently feather the skin from the center of the face outwards. This is another good TV accompanying activity.

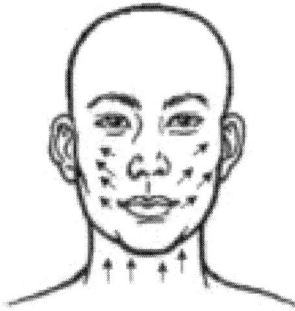

Correspondence Wanding

The ancient healers knew that if the left side of the body hurt you worked on the right. If the upper body hurt, you worked on the lower. Even today, some alternative health modalities will suggest working on the left knee if the right elbow is painful. There are all kinds of correspondences in the body.

Left knee/right elbow	Right knee/left elbow
Left ankle/right wrist	Right ankle/left wrist
Left little finger/right little	Right little finger/left little toe
Upper spine/lower belly	Upper chest/lower spine
Right shoulder/left hip	Left shoulder/right hip

Disease

Wanding

Techniques

Acne, Boils, Acne Rosacea

Micro-circulation is key to improving immune function and oxygenation of skin tissue. There are a couple of techniques that work with this condition.

The first technique is the cross-hatching technique much like drawing a tic-tac-toe game. Use the vertical motion first as it will draw energy up the face, then back down. It will restore any broken phase-locked scalar waves, break up congestion and toxins, improve microcirculation and wake up your lazy immune system. This technique also stimulates the elastin and collagen in the skin to improve skin texture. This can be done for about ten minutes, while you are watching your favorite movie or TV show.

The second technique is also a cross-hatching technique but the vertical and horizontal strokes are short and accordion-like, zig zagging up and down the face. The horizontal strokes also wiggle across the face in a short zigzag fashion. This tends to break up cystic acne and boils better than the straight cross-hatching technique. This can also be done for ten minutes or so.

The third technique is the circular clockwise movement that is quite calming and smooths out the energy. This is a good finishing technique when you have used the cross-hatching. This can be done for two to three minutes to calm the face.

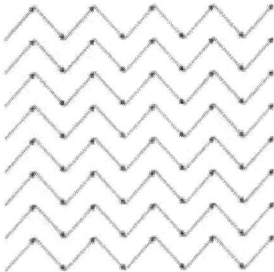

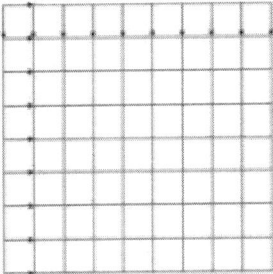

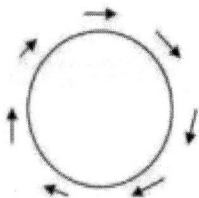

ADD, ADHD

Calming children and adult that have a hard time paying attention or who are hyperactive can be a challenge. Place your hand flat against the base of their neck with your fingers together. Just below where your lower finger touches the chest is where the thymus gland is located. Remember where that spot is and remove your hand.

Move the wand clockwise about once per second – one thousand and one, one thousand and two and so on – around the area of the thymus. You will notice their energy relax and they will become more calm. Other wanding patterns may be two intense and distracting so stick with the circular one over the thymus gland. The time needed for this technique varies, some children begin to calm quite quickly and some take a little longer.

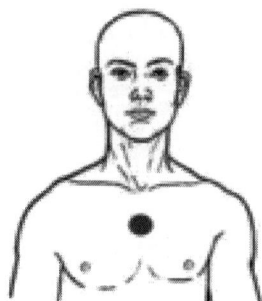

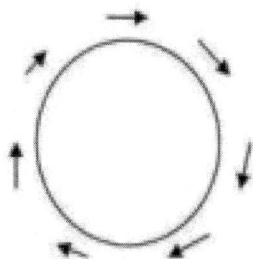

Anxiety

This technique can be self-administered or can be used on others. Place your hand flat against the base of the front of the neck with your fingers and thumb together. Just below where your lower finger touches the chest is where the thymus gland is located. Remember where that spot is and remove your hand.

Move the wand clockwise about once per second – one thousand and one, one thousand and two and so on – around the area of the thymus. You will notice the energy relax and a feeling of peace will blanket the mind and it will become more calm. Other wanding patterns may be two intense and distracting so stick with the circular one over the thymus gland. Ten to twenty minutes is a good time to start to see results.

Another technique if you are anxious is use the wand on a point on the bottoms of your feet. This point is located on the bottom of the foot, in the middle, just after the ball of the foot. You will feel it almost like a groove. Take the rounded tip of the wand and place it on the groove. This point helps move the overall qi and blood of the body and relieves a feeling of being stuck in whatever is going on in your life. Massage this point with the wand briskly with a light to medium rubbing action on both feet for about 30 seconds each. Repeat as often as necessary.

About three quarters of an inch below the knuckle of the first finger, towards the wrist, is a place where you can roll or rub to relieve anxiety also.

Another good point for calming anxiety is located right between the eyebrows, in the indentation between your forehead and the bridge of the nose. This point is also called the third eye. It helps calm the body and mind. Place the rounded tip of the wand softly on this point and roll the tip of the wand gently until you feel a shift.

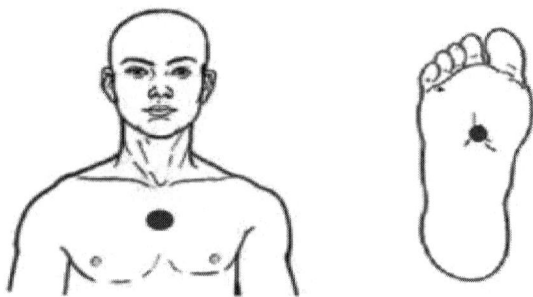

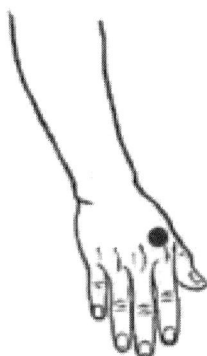

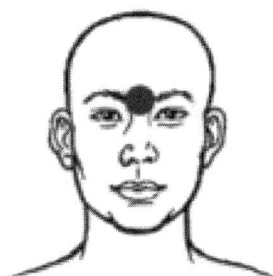

Inflammatory Arthritis, Rheumatism

As these conditions suggest they are the result of inflammation. Remember the house burning down scenario? These conditions are quite difficult to treat with even a good quality zero-point energy wand alone. You need to get to the root of the inflammation. It has been shown in research that inflammation usually results from a body that is overly acidic in addition to being dehydrated and is presenting free radical damage. While the zig zag cross hatching technique may help reduce your pain, until you get the inflammation under control with diet and supplementation, especially with high doses of antioxidants, you will probably not see significant improvement with the wand alone.

This would be a good place to mention that it has been discovered that 93% of the people in the USA are deficient in Vitamin D. Mayer Eisenstein, MD, JD, MPH spoke on *The Newly Rediscovered Anti-Aging Properties of the Amazing Sunshine Vitamin D* at the 16th annual A4M conference in Las Vegas, Nevada. Also discussed was the use of Vitamin D to increase protection from cancer, chronic pain, decrease falls, and possibly protect yourself from influenza. Dr. Einstein recommends 5000 IU's daily to his patients but he and his colleagues takes as much as 10,000 IU's a day. See this video on

YouTube.

http://www.youtube.com/watch?v=8wmb8B6E9RY

Remember to discuss with your primary care doctor what is best for you.

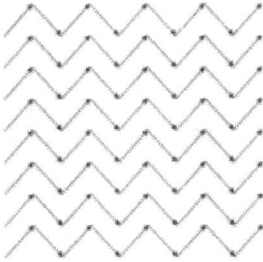

Osteoarthritis

This type of arthritis, responds better to a good quality zero-point energy wand than the inflammatory type. The best technique is a cross-hatching technique but the vertical and horizontal strokes are short and accordion-like, zig zagging up and down the sore spots. The horizontal strokes also wiggle across the sore area in a short zigzag fashion. This tends to break up the joint congestion better than the straight cross-hatching technique. It is also good for swelling.

The straight cross-hatching technique is also good for localized congestion and swelling and it entails moving the wand vertically and horizontally over the sore area.

Always finish with the circular clockwise movement of the wand doing one clockwise rotation per second – one thousand and one, one thousand and two- for about 30 seconds to a minute after the pain subsides.

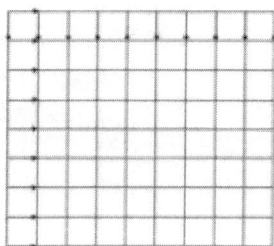

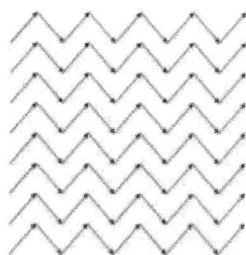

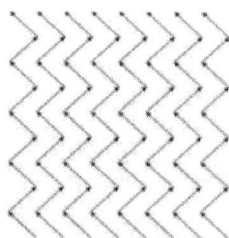

Ascites

Ascites is an accumulation of water in the peritoneal cavity. It can have various causes which can be medically significant. It is usually removed by aspirating it with a needle by a medical professional. You may get some relief by using a technique like dotting an I when writing. By tapping or dotting four times per second for about 30 seconds at each position around the abdomen, followed by the zigzag cross-hatching technique where you use a zigzagging pattern you can help break up the congestion.

Another technique for reducing the fluid build-up is to wand the back of the forearm. Look at the back of your hand. Starting from your wrist, stoke the line from the middle finger up to the mid-forearm. Slant the wand slightly so that you are using the side of the rounded tip. Lift the wand, return it to your wrist and stroke it up the forearm to the midpoint. Keep repeating.

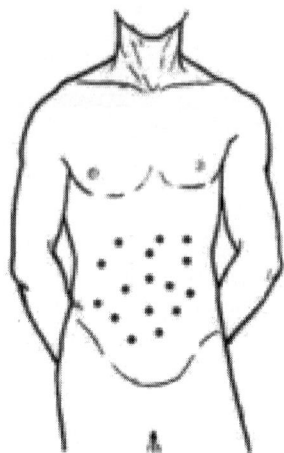

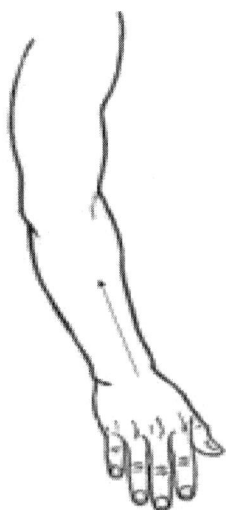

Asthma

Breathing problems can be very alarming as the wheezing, coughing and shortness of breath escalates. The only thing the zero-point energy wand can do with asthma is calm the body and reduce pain. The cross-hatching or zigzag cross-hatching over the thymus and bronchial tubes may bring some relief from congestion. The clockwise circular technique about one circle per second is very calming, may assist the labored breathing and help the medication work faster.

Another good wanding place that may relieve asthmatic symptoms is on the wrist. Turn your hand so that your hand is vertical with your thumb on top and your little finger on the bottom. Raise your thumb so that it is pointing up in the air. Place two finger widths against the base of your thumb. The place beside where your outside finger touches the skin is the place to use the rolling or rubbing technique on each wrist.

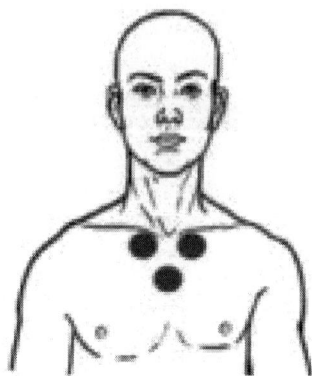

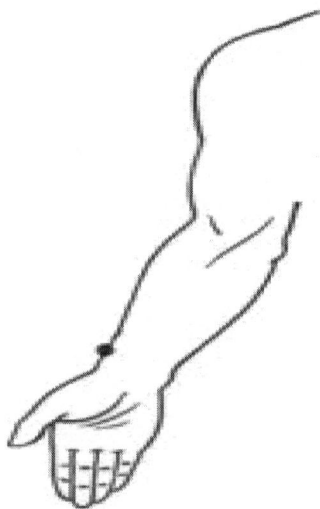

Back Pain

The best way to relieve back pain is to wand your feet. The chart on the next page shows where the spine is on the big toe side of the foot. Put the wand on the heel end of the spine section on the foot. pull the energy up the foot towards the big toe. Lift the wand off the foot, return to the toe end and pull the energy up again. Do it until you feel energized and your pain is reduced.

Another technique is to run your finger along the same place where the spine is on your foot until you find a sore spot, then place the tip of the wand on the sore spot and gently massage it until the pain releases.

If you want to use points elsewhere on your body to relieve back pain, there is a point on the inside of the leg (see image below), just below the knee. If you feel around, you will find a sore spot. Rub or roll that spot with the rounded end of the wand.

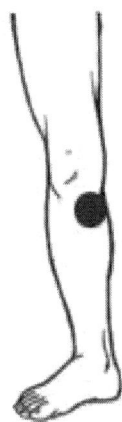

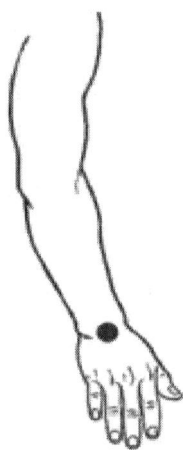

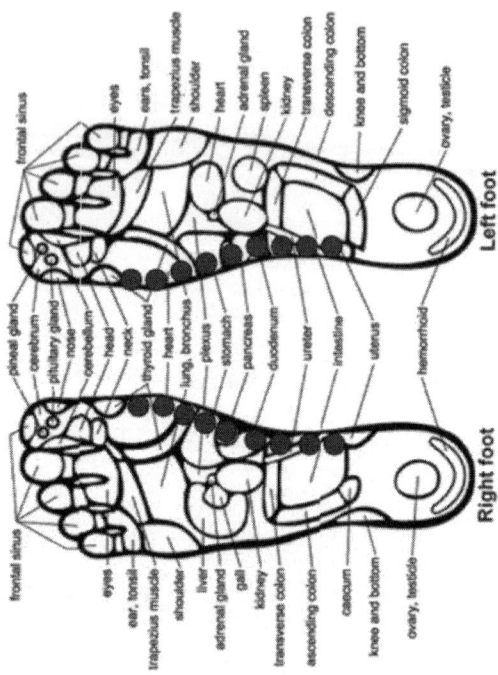

Left foot

frontal sinus
eyes
ears, tonsil
trapezius muscle
shoulder
heart
adrenal gland
spleen
kidney
transverse colon
descending colon
knee and bottom
sigmoid colon
ovary, testicle

Right foot

frontal sinus
eyes
ear, tonsil
trapezius muscle
shoulder
liver
adrenal gland
gall
kidney
transverse colon
ascending colon
caecum
knee and bottom
ovary, testicle

pineal gland
cerebrum
pituitary gland
nose
cerebellum
head
neck
thyroid gland
heart
lung, bronchus
plexus
stomach
pancreas
duodenum
ureter
intestine
uterus
haemorrhoid

46

Bell's Palsy

Bell's Palsy is something that seems to appear out of nowhere and can disappear just as fast. A good wanding place that may relieve the paralysis is on the wrist. Turn your hand so that your hand is vertical with your thumb on top and your little finger on the bottom. Raise your thumb so that it is pointing up in the air. Place two finger widths against the base of your thumb. The place beside where your outside finger touches the skin is the place to use the rolling or rubbing technique on each wrist.

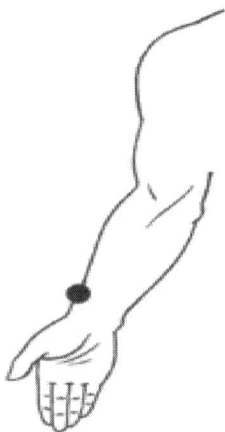

Broken Bones

Wanding through the cast to where the bone is broken can help the bone knit faster. Initially the cross-hatching or zigzag cross-hatching will help to reduce swelling and relieve congestion near the break site.

After the first 24 to 48 hours, you can use the stroking or the dotting technique, followed by the circular technique.

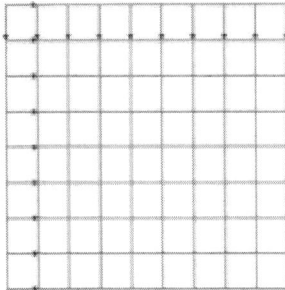

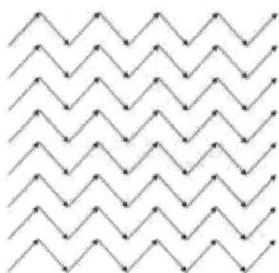

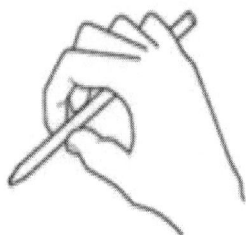

50

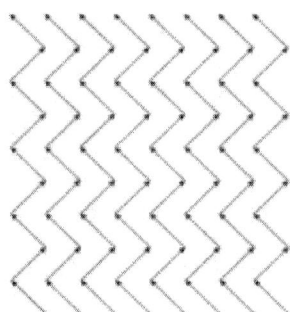

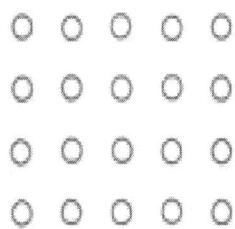

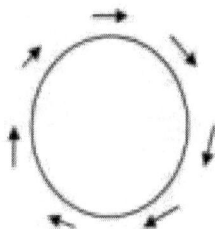

Bruises

As mentioned above, the side-brushing technique is excellent for bruising. It can also be used in conjunction with the cross-hatching technique or the zigzag cross-hatching technique if there is swelling along with the bruise.

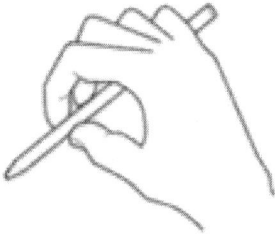

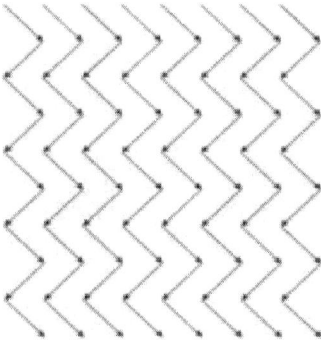

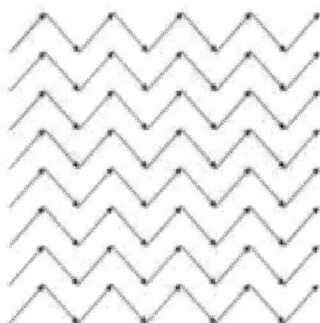

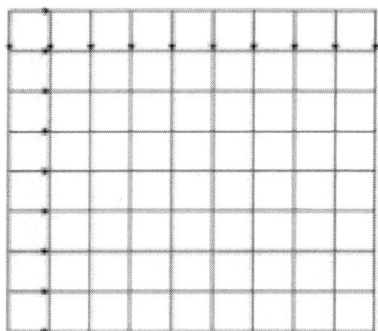

Cancer Pain

The pain from cancer can be quite difficult to bear. Not only is their anxiety, there is the anticipation of the pain. Any combination of the above techniques with the exception of the feathering, side-rolling and face-lifting techniques are all excellent for relieving pain. Try different techniques to see which ones work best.

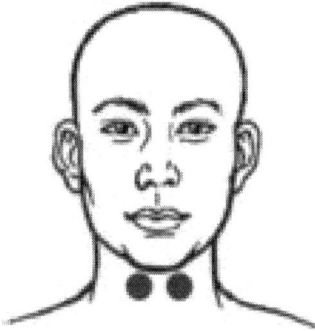

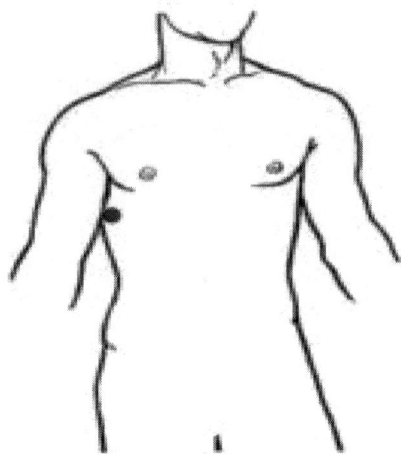

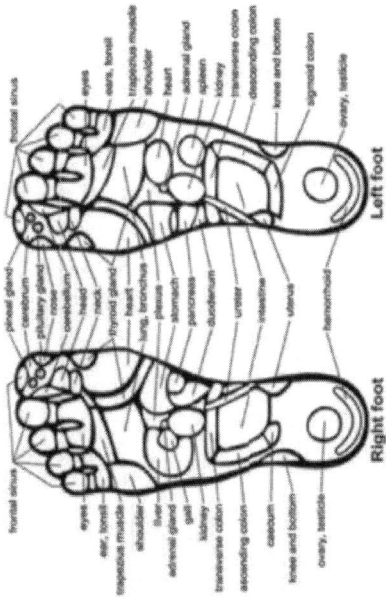

Left foot

Right foot

frontal sinus

eyes
ear, tonsil
trapezius muscle
shoulder
liver
gall
adrenal gland
kidney
transverse colon
descending colon
caecum
knee and bottom
ovary, testicle

pineal gland
cerebrum
pituitary gland
nose
cerebellum
neck
head
thyroid gland
lung, bronchus
heart
spleen
stomach
pancreas
duodenum
ureter
intestine
uterus
haemorrhoid

frontal sinus

eyes
ears, tonsil
trapezius muscle
shoulder
heart
adrenal gland
spleen
kidney
transverse colon
descending colon
knee and bottom
sigmoid colon
ovary, testicle

Carpal Tunnel Syndrome

57

The pain from Carpal Tunnel can be quite a problem, particularly at night. Most people with carpal tunnel syndrome know that you have to keep you hands and arms in a certain position to avoid the pain and numbness. That's not always possible at night. The swelling and information in the nerve channel needs to be alleviated and repaired so that it doesn't get worse.

Using the cross-hatching, zigzag cross-hatching, dotting, and directional dipping techniques on the inside of the wrists may help improve nerve transmission and blood supply.

You can also use a stroking motion from the wrist midline up to the middle of your forearm.

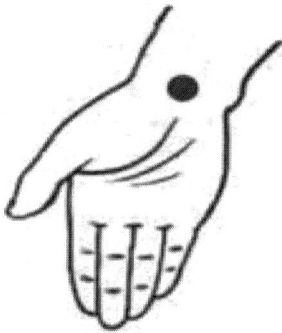

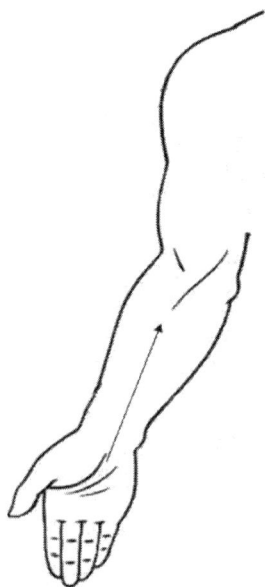

Early Onset Cirrhosis

Use the directional dipping or side rolling technique from the joint of the big toe to the inside side of the ankle.

You can also use any form of cross-hatching, ending with circling across your abdomen just below the ribs on the right hand side of your body.

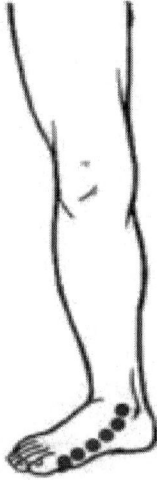

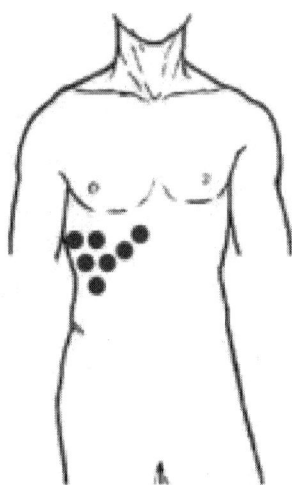

Cognitive Difficulties

Turn your hand so that your hand is vertical with your thumb on top and your little finger on the bottom. Raise your thumb so that it is pointing up in the air. Place two finger widths against the base of your thumb. The place beside where your outside finger touches the skin is the place to use the rolling or rubbing technique on each wrist.

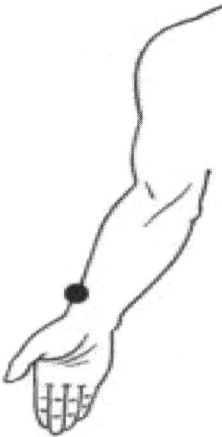

Colds

Behind your ears towards the back of your head, you will feel a bump on either side of your head. Wand those with dotting, circle dipping, tip tapping or any form of cross-hatching.

Another place you can wand with the same techniques is on the ankle. Imagine you see a clock face on the inside ankle. At 9 o'clock on the inside of the left ankle and 3 o'clock on the inside of the right ankle, about an inch out from your ankle you will feel a sore spot. Feel around until you find it. Wand each ankle with any of the techniques that we have listed.

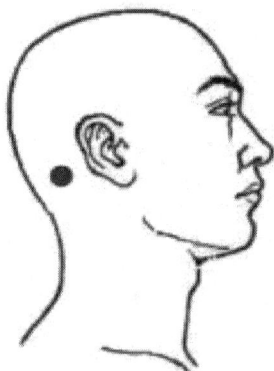

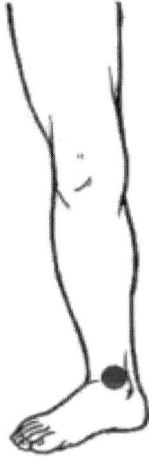

Colic

Colic is a digestive distress that can be alleviated by using any of the wanding techniques on the abdomen. Some babies get very severe colic that needs some of the more penetrating techniques such as dipping. Cross hatching may also work well, especially when wanding on babies tummy, to break up the inflammation, gas, gastric and intestinal disturbance.

One technique that could work very well for colic in babies is to wand in circles around their knees making sure you are wanding upwards on the inside of their knees.

Also for colic in babies there is a place on the back of the hand that you can wand which may help cramping. Bend your fingers so you can see your knuckles. On the knuckle of the first finger, is a spot just on the wrist edge of the knuckle on the babies hand which may relieve the cramping if you use a gentle rolling or rubbing technique there. You can also wand just above the skin on the hand.

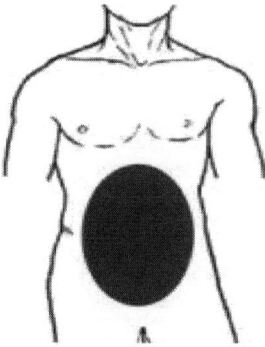

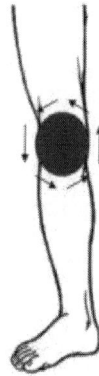

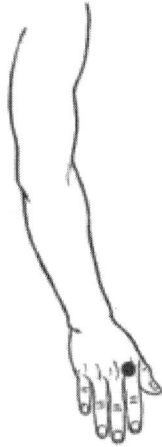

Colitis, Crohn's Disease, IBS

Wanding a spot at the back of the knee in the center of the crease where the knee bends can be quite effective for digestive upsets. Use whatever technique feels comfortable, although the rolling technique is one we suggest.

The knuckle of the first finger is a good place to do the circling technique. Keep the clockwise circles small enough to just encompass the outer edge of the bones.

One technique that could work very well for digestive discomfort is to wand in circles around your knees making sure you are wanding upwards on the inside of your knees.

For digestive upsets there is a place on the back of your hand that you can wand which may help cramping and diarrhea. Bend your fingers so you can see your knuckles. Two finger widths from the knuckle towards the wrist, is a spot that if you use the rolling technique or the rubbing technique may relieve your cramping and diarrhea.

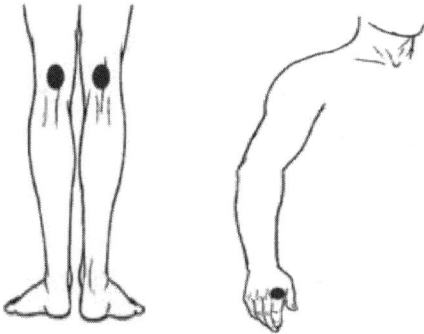

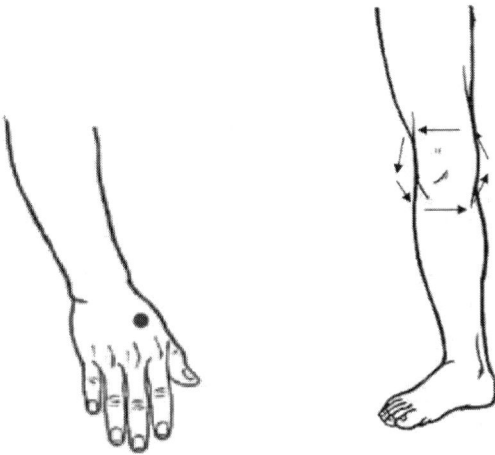

Constipation

There are a few places you can wand for constipation. One is on the foot, in the center, just below the ball. Use the rubbing or rolling technique with medium pressure.

The other place you can wand in on your hand . Look at the back of your hand with your fingers straight and together. Extend your thumb sideways at right angles to your fingers. Two finger widths in from the edge of the webbing between your thumb and your first finger you will feel the soft fleshy part next to a bone. If you can feel the bone with the tip of your finger you are in the right place. Use the rubbing or rolling technique there for a few minutes.

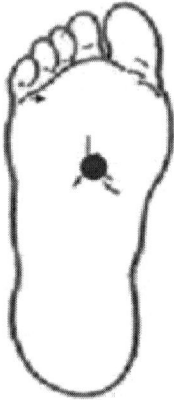

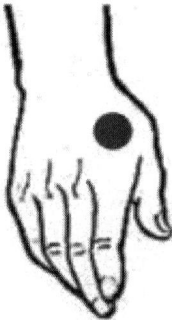

Coughing

One of the best controls for coughing is to reach about a handwidth below the armpit on the right side of the body then feel around for a sore spot with your thumb. If you put your arm down by your side, it is in line with the front of your arm. Put the tip of the wand on the spot and use the rubbing or rolling technique. The left side is for something else, so don't use it for cough.

Another good wanding place that may relieve coughing is on the wrist. Turn your hand so that your hand is vertical with your thumb on top and your little finger on the bottom. Raise your thumb so that it is pointing up in the air. Place two finger widths against the base of your thumb. The place beside where your outside finger touches the skin is the place to use the rolling or rubbing technique on each wrist.

Where the neck joins the spine there is a change in the bone. You may notice it as a lump. That is another good place to roll or rub the wand to relieve coughing.

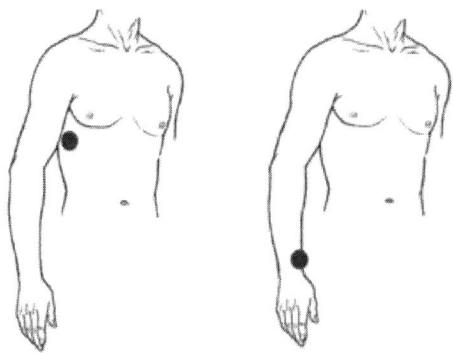

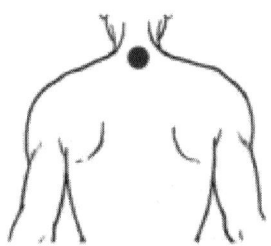

Cutaneous Vasculitis

Using the side brushing, tip tapping, directional dipping, circle dipping, or any of the cross-hatching techniques will help reduce the inflammation and restore the microcirculation. The more you can stimulate the micro-circulation, the more relief you will feel.

Also picking a spot where the cutaneous vasculitis is the worst and wanding there will help improve the blood circulation throughout the body. The blood makes a complete circuit throughout the body every four minutes.

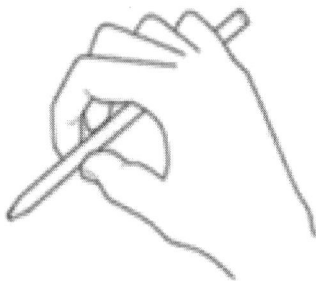

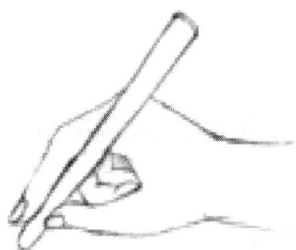

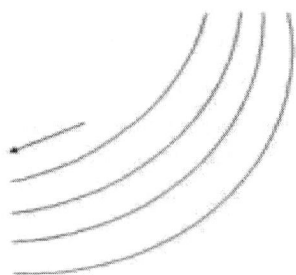

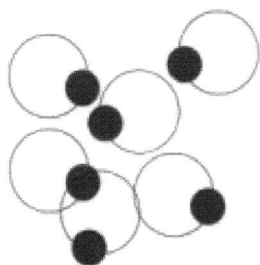

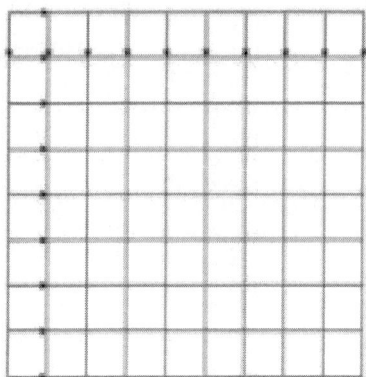
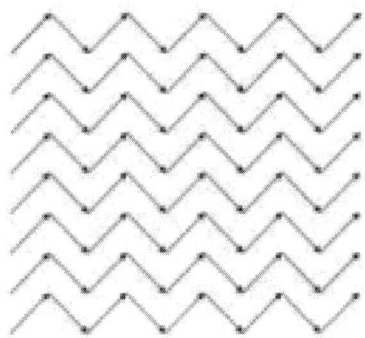

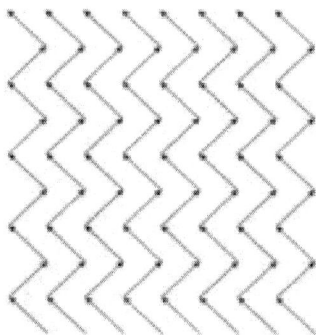

Cuts and Scrapes, Surgical Wounds

Wanding the wound site with a cross-hatching, zigzag cross-hatching, directional dipping, and the clockwise circular motion will help speed healing and restore circulation.

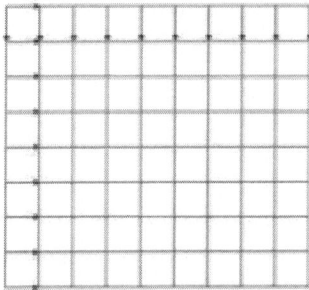

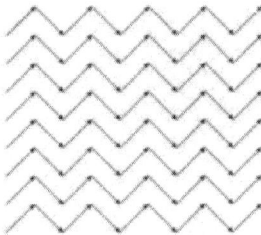

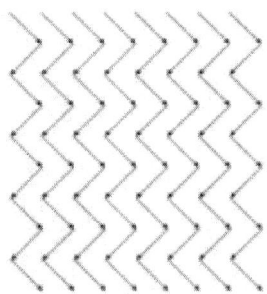

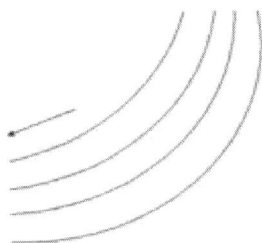

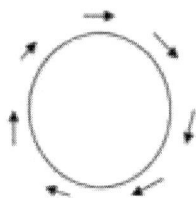

Dermatitis, Eczema, Psoriasis

Using the long stroking technique, stroke your wand from the base of your wrist on the back of your hand, up to the mid-forearm. Lift the wand up and return it to the base of the wrist to begin the next stroke.

If the skin is not too itchy and irritated you can use a side-brushing technique right on top of your skin problem.

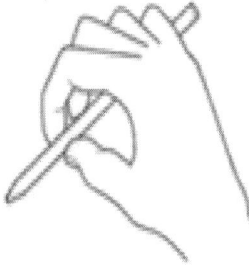

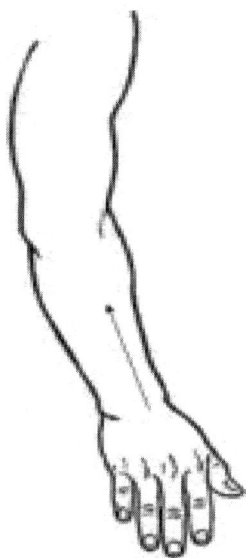

Diabetes

Bend one of your elbows and pinch the fleshy part of the elbow on the outside of your arm. Where your thumb rests on the fleshy part, use the rolling or rubbing technique. You can follow it up with the clockwise circular motion. Be sure to do both arms.

Also roll or rub the joint at the base of the thumb with the rolling, rubbing or circular techniques.

Look at your thumb with the thumb nail facing you. Wand the skin on the right hand edge of where the nail meets the skin using the rubbing technique.

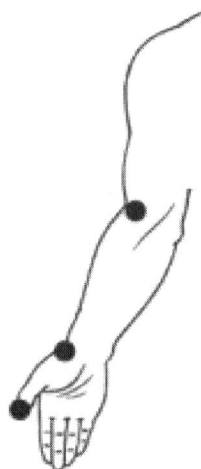

Energy Boost

There are some cross-road points that are really good for boosting your energy. These points are where more than one energy pipeline meet or cross one another. The first one is where the neck meets the spine. There is a lump of bone there and if you poke at it, it may be sore. You may be able to reach it with the wand and use the rubbing technique there. If you can't reach it, get someone to do the rolling technique for you.

The next spot that helps to boost energy is on the inside of the leg, just above the ankle. The rubbing, rolling or directional dipping techniques work well here.

Another place that is good for energy boosting is on the wrist. Turn your hand so than your thumb is facing up and your little finger is facing down. Lift your thumb so that it is vertical. Lay three fingers against the base of your thumb. Where your first finger rests on the skin, directly in line with the thumb is where you will use the rolling or rubbing technique.

The next place is one hands width below the armpit on the left side of the body. You will find a place directly in line with your arm if it was by your side that will be sore if you poke at it. If you bend your left arm you should be able to feel the spot with your thumb. Use the rolling technique there.

If you wand a two to three inch diameter circle on the top of the head right where the 'soft' spot used to be soft, it will draw your energy up your body and give you a needed boost.

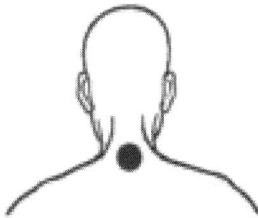

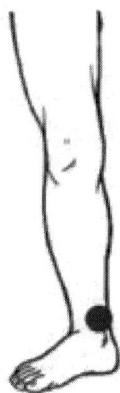

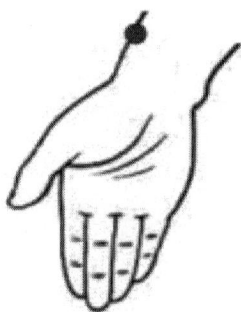

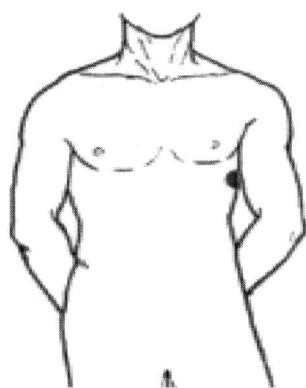

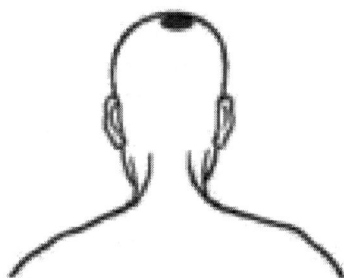

Eye Problems

Use the clockwise circular wanding motion over and around the eyes to improve microcirculation and help relieve eye problems.

Using firm pressure, use a stroking technique from the knuckle of your first finger up to your wrist. Lift the wand and return to the starting point to continue.

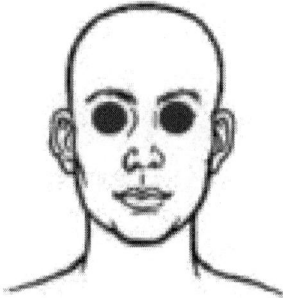

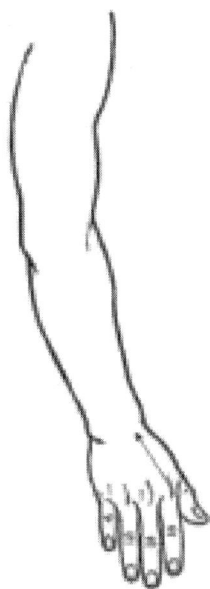

Fatigue

Using a back and forth stroking technique on the outside of each knee from the top of the kneecap to the bottom of the kneecap will give you more energy so you feel less fatigued. You may have to repeat this wanding process several times to notice a result.

With your palm facing you there is a little bump of bone on the little finger side of the hand, where the hand meets the wrist. Use the wand in a clockwise circular motion, rubbing the outside of the bone, in addition to the lump of bone itself.

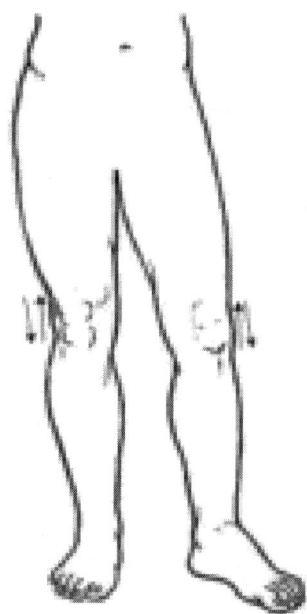

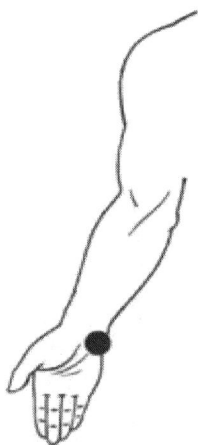

Fat Loss

To jump start and rev up your metabolism, reach about a hand-width below the armpit on the left side of the body then feel around for a sore spot with your thumb. If you put your arm down by your side, it is in line with the front of your arm. Put the tip of the wand on the spot and use the rubbing or rolling technique. The right side is for something else, so don't use it for fat loss.

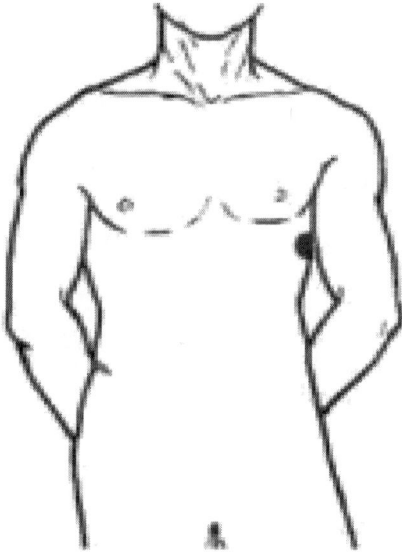

Fibromyalgia (See also Trigger Points)

A good technique for general all-over body pain, is reach about a handwidth below the armpit then feel around for a sore spot with your thumb. If you put your arm down by your side, it is in line with the front of your arm. Put the tip of the wand on the spot and use the rubbing or rolling technique.

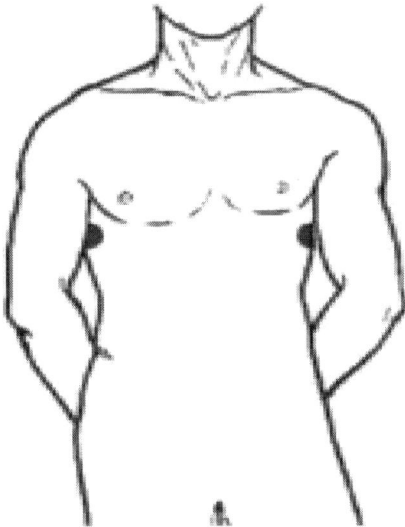

Fine Lines and Wrinkles

The side brushing, feathering and side-rolling techniques work well for fine lines and wrinkles anywhere on the body. The wanding process improves the microcirculation in the skin thus improving elastin and collagen production and maintenance.

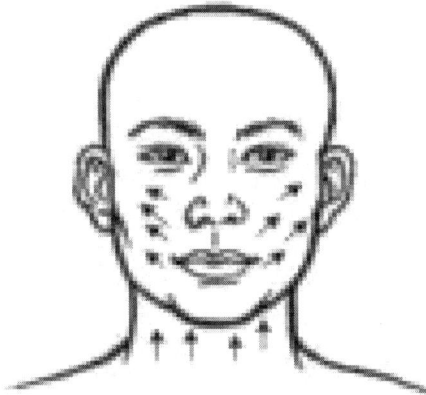

Flu

Behind your ears towards the back of your head, you will feel a bump on either side of your head. Wand those with dotting, circle dipping, tip tapping or any form of cross-hatching.

Another place you can wand with the same techniques is on the outside of the ankle. Imagine you see a clock face on the inside ankle. At 2 o'clock, on a clock face, about an inch from your right ankle, and 10 o'clock on your left ankle, you will feel a sore spot. Feel around until you find it. Wand each ankle with any of the techniques that we have listed under the flu category.

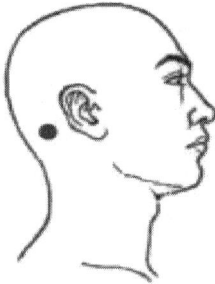

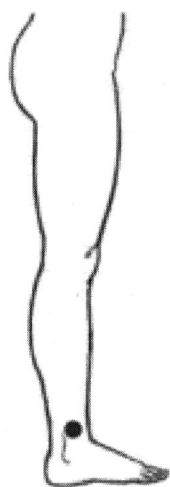

Fuzzy Thinking

Look at the palm of your hand. On your little finger side of your hand you will notice a bump of bone at the wrist crease. Use the rolling or rubbing technique there often.

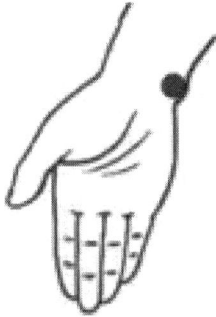

GERD

This is the fancy name for heartburn. Using a back and forth stroking technique on the outside of each knee from the top of the kneecap to the bottom of the kneecap will help relieve your discomfort. You may have to repeat this wanding process several times to notice that your heartburn has not returned.

Also you may find a sore spot about two inches above the inside of your ankle. Feel around for it. You can use the rolling or rubbing technique, followed always by the clockwise circling technique to relieve your heartburn as well. These two places work well together.

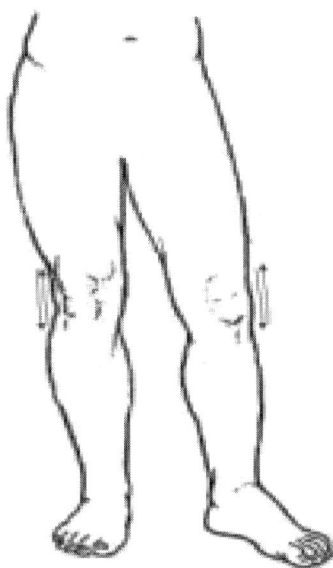

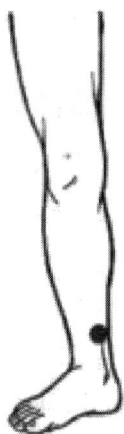

Gingivitis

Reduce the pain and inflammation with the circling, directional dipping, tip tapping or rubbing techniques to improve circulation and stimulate immune response. Wand on the cheeks following the line of the teeth and gums.

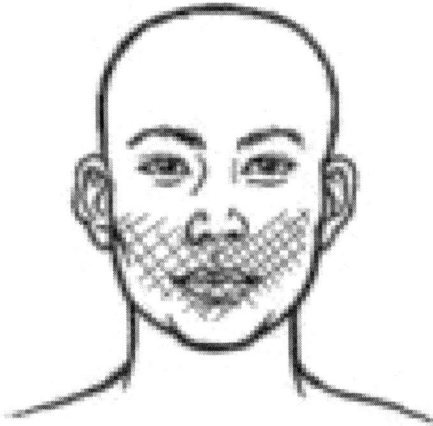

Gout

The circle dipping, circling and cross-hatching techniques work really well on-site for gout. Gout typically affects the big toe and it can be extremely painful. Wherever it hurts is where you wand it.

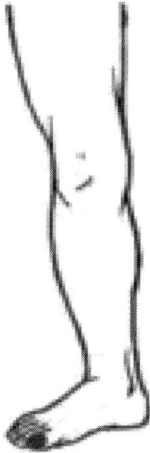

Headaches, Migraines

Headaches particularly migraines can plague people for days. Try this technique and see if you get some relief. Turn your hand vertically so that your thumb is on the top, your little finger is on the bottom and your palm is on the side. Lift your thumb so that it is sticking up. Place two fingers against your raised thumb on your wrist. Stick your wand on the spot by your outside finger on top of your arm and use the rubbing or rolling technique there. Do the spot on the other arm.

Another good place to wand, especially for migraines is the temples. Using the circle or circle dotting technique is the most soothing and calming.

Behind the ears towards the back of the head is a bump. This area is another good headache reliever. Use the rubbing, rolling or circular technique here.

Wanding the top of the head in a clockwise circular motion can relieve the pressure of a headache.

Also wanding the knuckle of the first finger can provide some relief from headaches. You can also rub or roll the wand in the webbing of the thumb, being sure to use the wand right up against the bones.

114

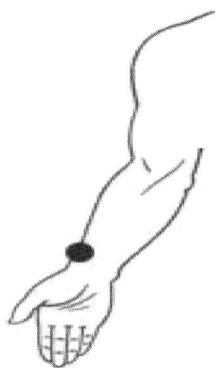

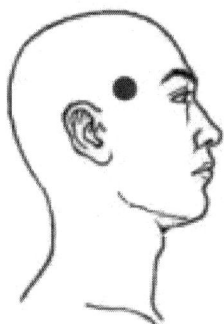

115

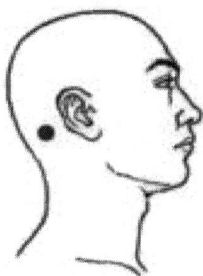

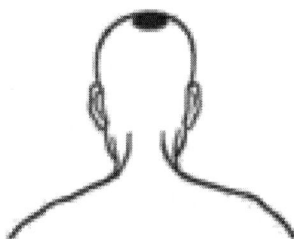

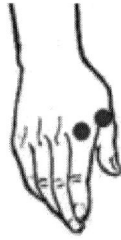

Heart Pain, Heart Palpitations

This is not something to fool around with. This is an emergency technique until you can get medical help. Look at your hand with the palm facing you. At the base of your hand where you see a crease where it joins the arm, find the midline. Place your finger in the place just beside the midline, towards your thumb. Stick the tip of the wand beside your finger and use the rolling technique with medium pressure on this spot.

On the inside of the wrist, three finger widths up from the crease in the wrist, is another place you can wand until help arrives using the rubbing or rolling technique.

You can also wand the bump at the wrist crease on the little finger side of the hand with a circular technique, making contact with the skin.

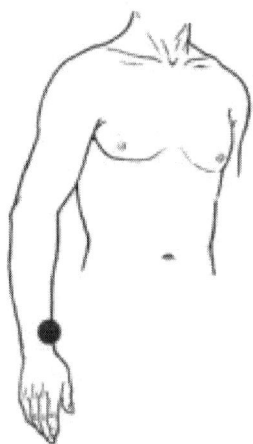

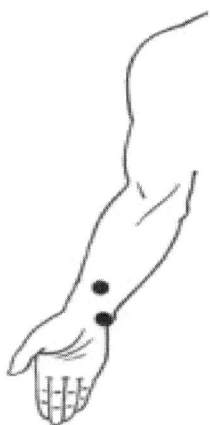

Hemorrhoids

It is kind of hard to wand your butt and it may be something you only want to do in very familiar company. So to be discreet about what is going on, it is best to wand points on the bottoms of your feet that correspond to the rectum.

There is another point on the arm you can use to reduce the pain and swelling. Turn your hand perpendicular to the floor with your thumb on the top and your little finger on the bottom. Raise your thumb so that it is sticking straight up in the air. Place your hand on your are against your thumb with your fingers and thumb beside each other. Estimate another three fingers up your arm. On a line in line with your thumb you will feel an indentation. Place the wand there and use the rolling technique to help your butt feel better.

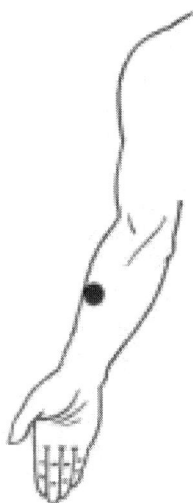

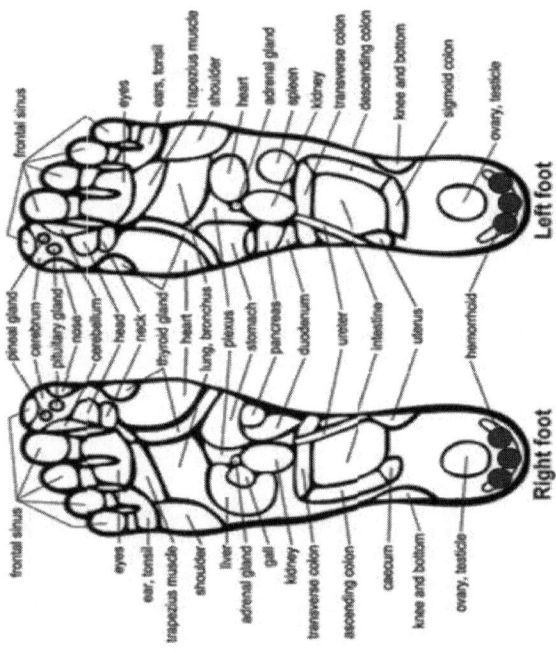

Left foot — frontal sinus, eyes, ears, tonsil, trapezius muscle, shoulder, heart, adrenal gland, spleen, kidney, transverse colon, descending colon, knee and bottom, sigmoid colon, ovary, testicle, uterus, intestine, ureter, duodenum, pancreas, stomach, plexus, lung, bronchus, heart, thyroid gland, neck, cerebellum, head, nose, pituitary gland, cerebrum, pineal gland

Right foot — frontal sinus, eyes, ear, tonsil, trapezius muscle, shoulder, liver, adrenal gland, gall, kidney, transverse colon, ascending colon, caecum, knee and bottom, ovary, testicle, haemorrhoid

122

Herpes, Shingles, Cold Sores

These can be very nasty conditions to get rid of and they can hang around and go dormant. Pain management with the wand is probably the best you can do without adding alternative treatment. Wand the area with cross-hatching, directional dipping and circular techniques.

In addition, you can wand a spot a hand's width down from the base of the throat in the center of the chest with any of the suggested wanding patterns for herpes, shingles and cold sores.

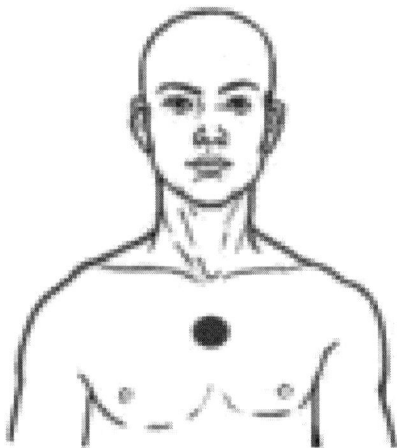

High Blood Pressure

Behind your ears towards the back of your head, you will feel a bump on either side of your head. Wand those with dotting, circle dipping, tip tapping or any form of cross-hatching.

Another place you can wand is on the top of the foot. Use the stroking technique from the base of the big toe to the place where there is a bump on the top of the foot in line with the big toe. Lift the wand and again, place it at the base of the big toe and pull it up to the base of the leg. Keep repeating and wand the other foot.

Bend your elbow and position your hand so that your thumb is at the top and your little finger is on the bottom. Two finger widths down from the crease in your elbow, in line with the thumb is a place where you can roll or rub the wand to help your high blood pressure.

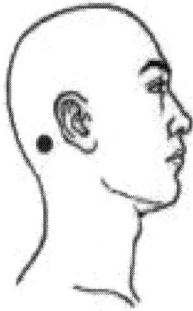

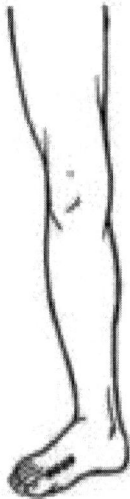

126

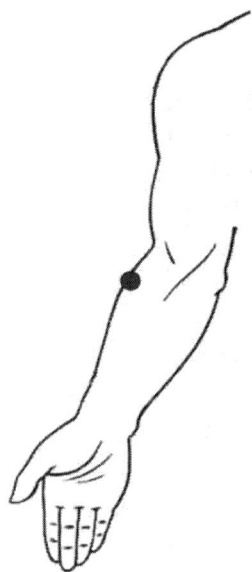

Hip Problems

Use any of the cross-hatching techniques and circular techniques on the hip directly. For deep rooted pain you can use the tip tapping, dotting, circle dipping and dipping techniques.

You might also want to try a place behind each knee. Right in the middle of the knee crease in the back of the knee use the rolling or rubbing technique to relieve pain.

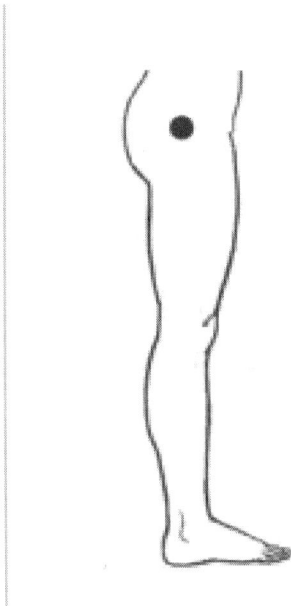

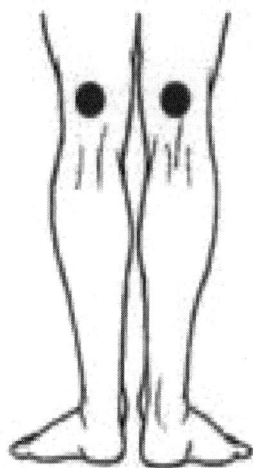

Impotence

Aside from wanding the obvious, there are a couple of places that you can wand that may help. Find the waist band of your slacks. Reach around to feel your back bone. Each side of the backbone, is the place where you wand using the rolling or rubbing technique.

The other place is on the inside of the ankle. Imagine you see a clock face there. At 10 o'clock about three quarters of an inch from the ankle bone on the left foot and 2 o'clock on the right foot, is where you use the rolling or rubbing technique.

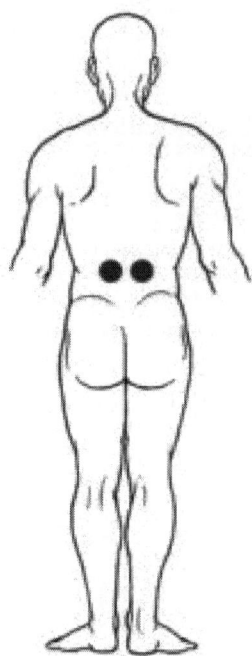

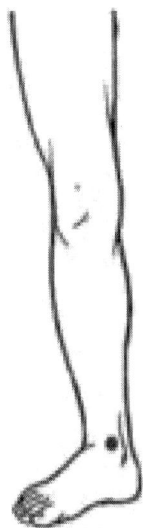

Improved Complexion

The face-lifting, side-rolling and side-brushing techniques are excellent for the face, helping to stimulate microcirculation, collagen and elastin production which helps to smooth out fine lines and wrinkles.

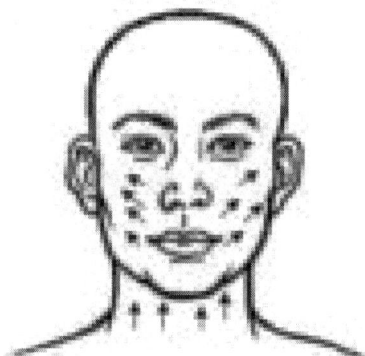

Insomnia, Sleeping Problems

The best technique for sleep really isn't one. All you have to do is put the wand on your beside table with the rounded end pointed at your pillow. If you are particularly wound up you can wand the anxiety place (see anxiety) with your wand before putting it on your bedside table.

Another technique is to use the rolling or rubbing technique on the thumb joints at the base of the thumb and on the bump on the little finger side of the hand where the hand joins the arm. And the final point at 10 o'clock on the left ankle and 2 o'clock on the right ankle.

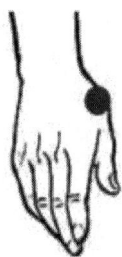

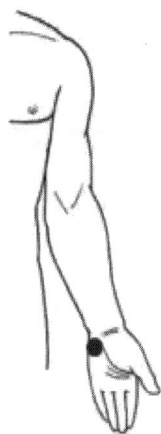

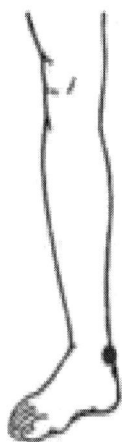

Iritis

Inflammation and infections in the eye can be extremely painful and irritating. Bend your arm at the elbow and cross-hatch a four inch square of skin from the crease of each elbow on the outside of your forearm.

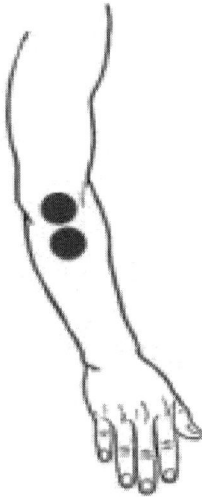

Early Onset Kidney Disease

If you have someone who can help you, get them to wand your kidney areas with the dipping, dotting, circle dipping and the cross-hatching techniques.

If you are doing this yourself the best technique is to wand a place on the bottoms of your feet. There is a place in the midline of your foot just between the arch and the ball of your foot. Use the rolling or rubbing technique there.

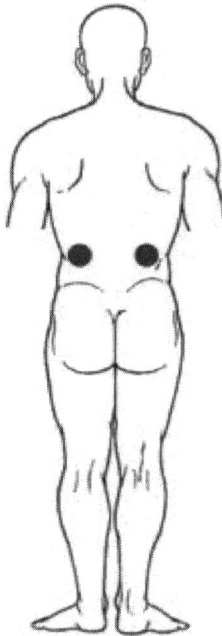

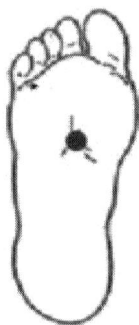

Knee Problems

All sorts of knee problems can be wanded. Most knee problems respond to wanding on the outside of the knee from the top center to the bottom center. You can touch the knee surface or you can wand one-half inch above it. You can also do any of the cross-hatching techniques, or circular techniques around the knee.

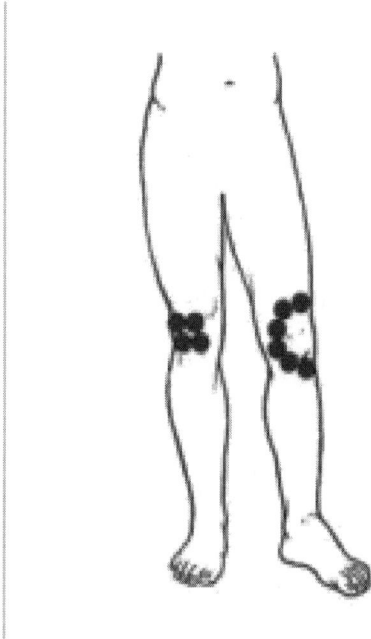

Macular Degeneration

About three finger widths from the foot end of the big toe, along the midline of the big toe, is the place to wand using the rubbing or rolling technique.

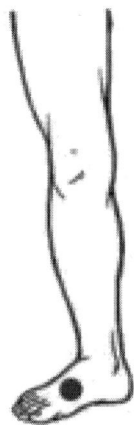

Motion Sickness

There are a couple of points that are very effective for motion sickness. One is on the wrist and one is on the bottoms of the feet. Look at the crease on the inside of your wrist where the hand meets the arm. Two finger widths from the crease in the middle of your wrist, you will feel an indentation. Place the rounded tip of the wand there. Use the rubbing or rolling technique for about a minute on each wrist or longer if you are still queasy.

The foot technique is also very effective. Find the spot on the picture below and use the rubbing or rolling technique for about a minute on each foot. You can increase the time if necessary.

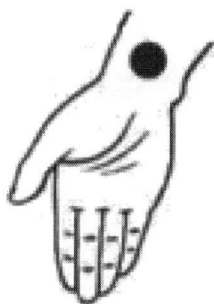

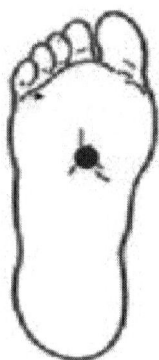

Multiple Sclerosis

Since multiple sclerosis is a degenerative disease, any technique that can slow the progression of it is a good thing. Wanding the head, neck and spine with a circle, circle dipping, dipping, directional dipping or dotting technique may help.

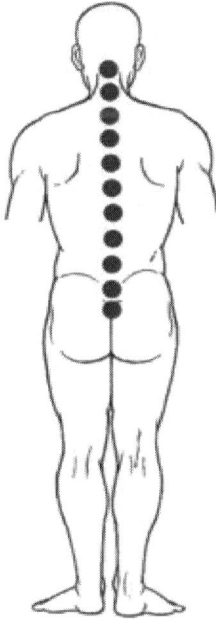

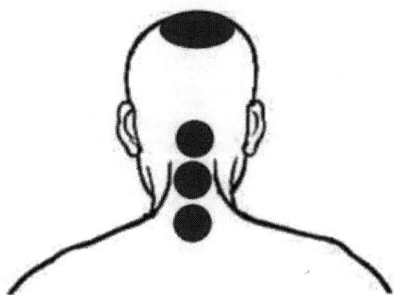

Muscle Spasms

Wand the area of the spasm with a dipping or circle dipping technique.

Another place you could wand for muscles spasms regardless of where they are is on the outside of the knee about one inch below the knee. Wand an inch wide band of skin from the bottom edge of the kneecap to the back of the knee, using a stroking technique.

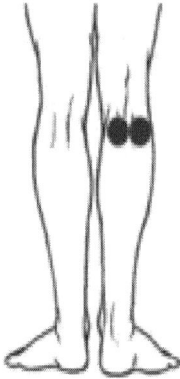

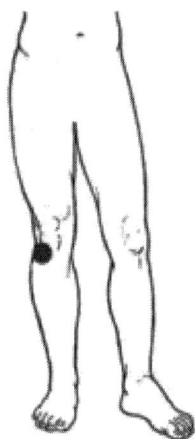

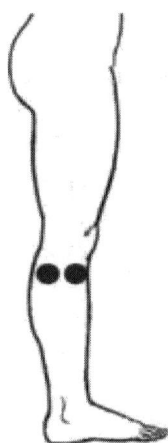

150

Muscle Strain

Working on location with muscle strains is best. To repair stretched and torn muscle fibers use the dipping, circle dipping, dotting, tip tapping or any cross-hatching technique so that it penetrates to the depth of the muscle.

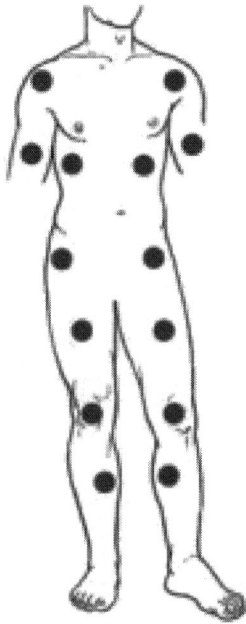

Nausea

There are a couple of points that are very effective for nausea. One is on the wrist and one is on the bottoms of the feet. If you can imagine that you have a string tied around your wrist where the hand meets the arm. Now look on the inside of the wrist where the string would be. In the middle of the inside of your wrist, you will feel an indentation. Place the rounded tip of the wand there. Use the rubbing or rolling technique for about a minute on each wrist.

The foot technique is also very effective. Find the spot on the picture below and use the rubbing or rolling technique for about a minute on each foot. Repeat at necessary.

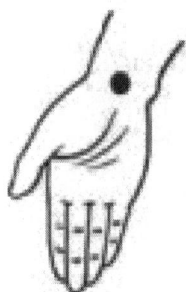
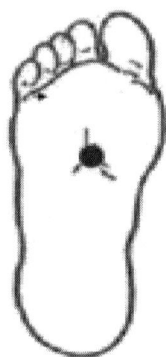

Neck Pain

Wanding the neck where it hurts is the first step. Any of the cross-hatching techniques, dotting, circle dipping or directional dipping followed by clockwise circling work well for neck pain.

Another place to relieve pain in the neck is on the bottom of the feet. Where the joint of the big toe is on the side of the foot is a where the neck points are. Dotting, tip tapping, rolling and rubbing are good techniques for this point.

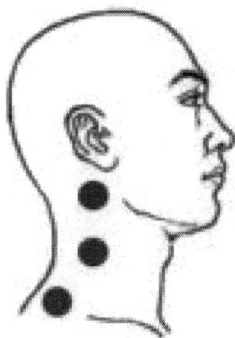

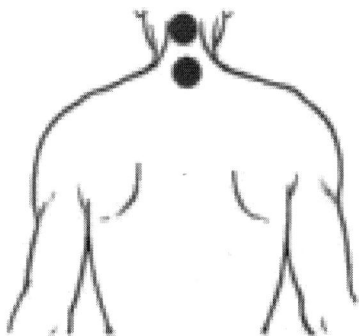

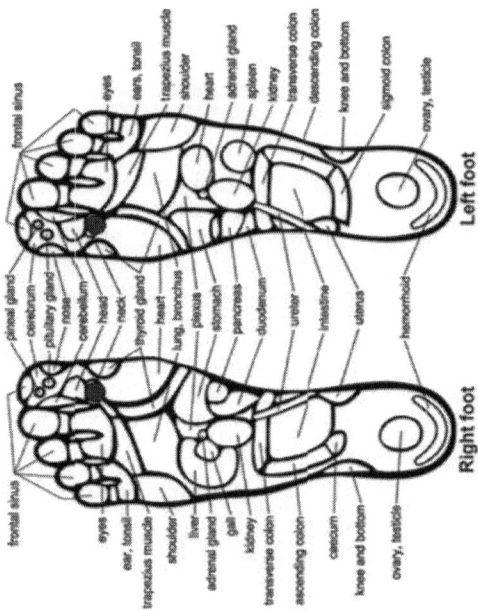

frontal sinus
eyes
ears, tonsil
trapezius muscle
shoulder
heart
adrenal gland
spleen
kidney
transverse colon
descending colon
knee and bottom
sigmoid colon
ovary, testicle

Left foot

pineal gland
cerebrum
pituitary gland
nose
cerebellum
head
neck
thyroid gland
heart
lung, bronchus
plexus
stomach
pancreas
duodenum
ureter
intestine
uterus
haemorrhoid

frontal sinus
eyes
ear, tonsil
trapezius muscle
shoulder
liver
adrenal gland
gall
kidney
transverse colon
ascending colon
caecum
knee and bottom
ovary, testicle

Right foot

158

Neuralgia

Using a rolling or rubbing technique at the sight of the pain can give relief.

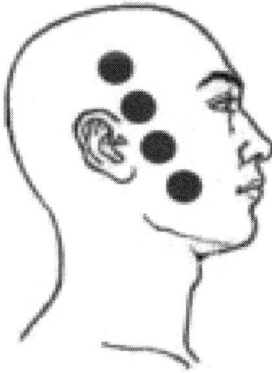

Neuropathy

Wanding the hip joint with a circle dipping, dipping, dotting, rolling, rubbing or tip tapping technique followed by the circular technique can help neuropathy, especially if it is combined with three other wanding sites. The first is on the outside of the knee at the midline. Use any of the above techniques to wand this area. The second place is a hand width above the ankle bone, in the midline, where you can do any of these techniques as well. The final place is a hand width above the ankle on the inside of the leg.

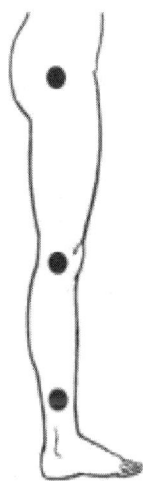

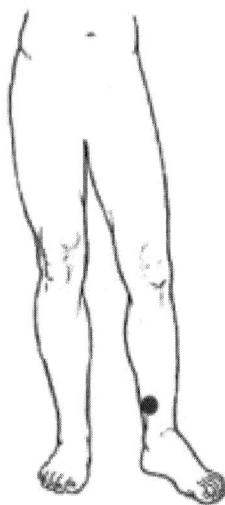

161

Osteoporosis

There are a couple of places where wanding may ease the pain. The first is along the spine. Use long strokes from the base of the spine to the neck just above the skin surface. You can follow that by circling.

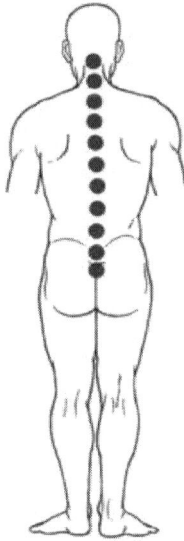

The next place is on the bottoms of the feet in the midline of the foot, between the ball of the foot and the arch. You will feel a slight indent there. Roll or rub the wand on that spot.

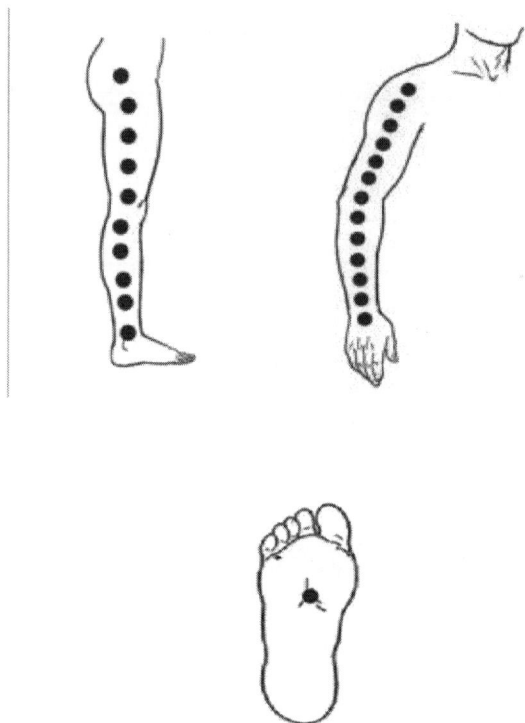

Pain

General and acute pain can be wanded by wanding on either side of the voice box from the neck under the chin to the base of the neck. Use a circular or circle dipping technique.

Another useful technique for general pain is a point under each armpit. Reach about a handwidth below the armpit then feel around for a sore spot with your thumb. If you put your arm down by your side, it is in line with the front of your arm. Put the tip of the wand on the spot and use the rubbing or rolling technique.

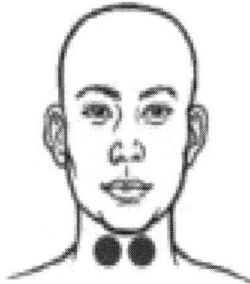

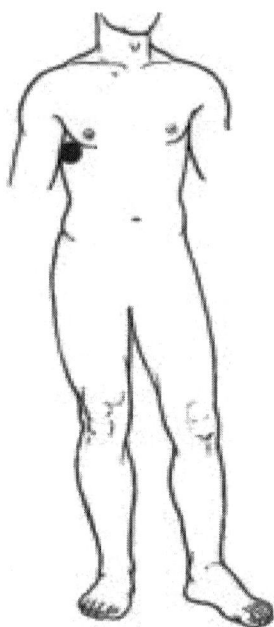

Panic Attacks

Wanding the base of the skull down to the base of the neck with a circular or stroking technique can sometimes relieve the escalating onset.

Here is another technique you might like. Place your hand flat against the base of the front of the neck with your fingers and thumb together. Just below where your lower finger touches the chest is where the thymus gland is located. Remember where that spot is and remove your hand.

Move the wand clockwise about once per second – one thousand and one, one thousand and two and so on – around the area of the thymus. You will notice the energy relax and a feeling of peace will blanket the mind and it will become more calm. Other wanding patterns may be two intense and distracting so stick with the circular one over the thymus gland. Ten to twenty minutes is a good time to start to see results.

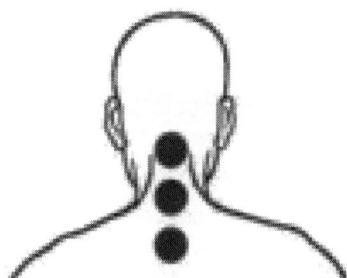

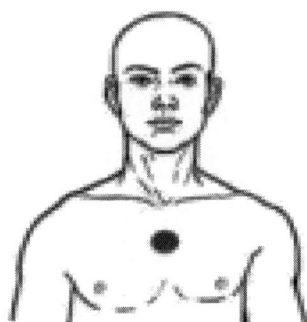

Plantar Fasciitis

Find the center of the calf muscle on the back of your leg. Use a rubbing or rolling technique in a golf ball sized area of the center of the calf, a hand width down from the back of the knee.

You can also wand the bottoms of the feet in a dipping or cross-hatching pattern from the heel to the ball of the foot.

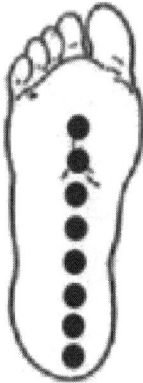

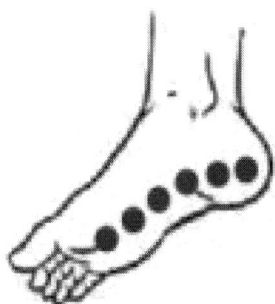

PMS

To relieve the symptoms of PMS and menstrual discomfort, stoke a zero-point energy wand from your pubic bone to your navel back and forth. This is also good to relieve the accompanying fatigue.

Also you may find a sore spot about two inches above the inside of your ankle. Feel around for it. You can use the rolling or rubbing technique, followed always by the clockwise circling technique.

Two other feet points are at 11 o'clock just behind the ankle on the left foot and 1 o'clock just behind the right ankle and a point on the top of the foot, where there is a bump of bone about the middle. Use the rubbing, rolling and side brushing techniques to relieve your discomfort and fatigue.

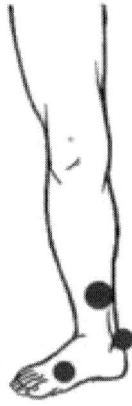

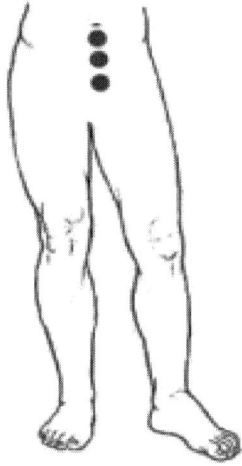

173

Reynaud's Disease

Wanding the elbows by touching the skin and circling the elbows may help prevent the onset of Reynaud's in the hands.

The other place to work with Reynaud's is at the base of the neck in the front of your body. If you feel around on the front of the base of your neck you will feel bones. Find the midline of your neck, then move two inches or so either side of your neck. You will feel a sore spot where this place is. Feel around for it. Use the rubbing or rolling technique there.

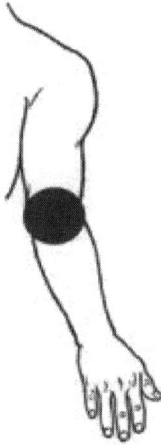

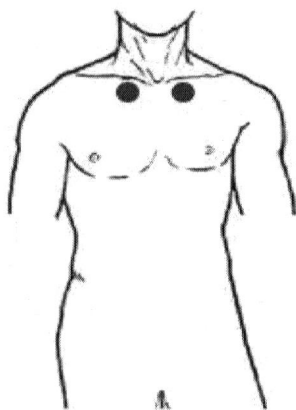

Rhinitis, Sinusitis

Find the place on the top of the head where babies have that soft spot. In adults, it sometimes feels like there is a bit of an indent in the head. By wanding that spot with any version of the cross-hatching, dipping, dotting, and/or circular motion, you can relieve pressure in the nose and sinuses.

Wanding the face with any of the above techniques will can also do the same thing.

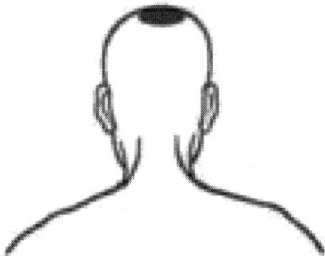

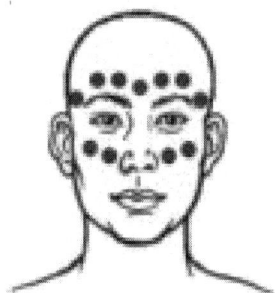

Sciatica

Sciatica pain can be wanded on location but be aware that the pain may travel so you will need to follow the pain with your wanding. It may travel right down the leg and into the foot. Use the circle dipping, circle dotting, directional dipping or either of the cross-hatching techniques.

Another technique involves wanding the bottoms of the heels of the feet. About one inch from the back of the bottom of the heel is a strip, about a finger width wide that goes from side to side. This is the sciatic part of the foot and it may be helpful to use a rubbing technique there.

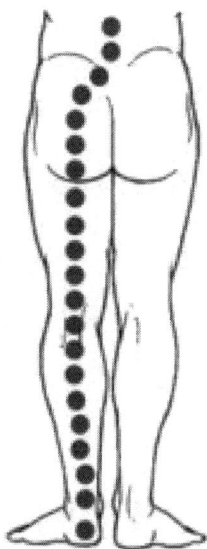

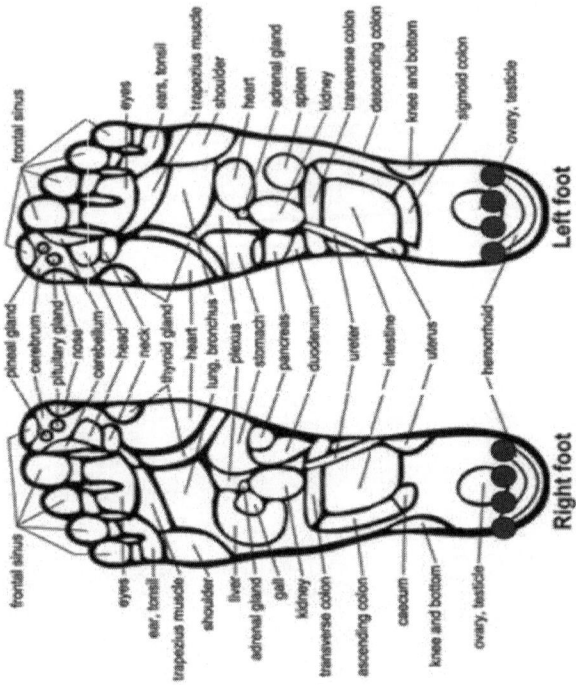

Left foot

Right foot

frontal sinus
eyes
ear, tonsil
trapezius muscle
shoulder
heart
adrenal gland
spleen
kidney
transverse colon
descending colon
knee and bottom
sigmoid colon
ovary, testicle

pineal gland
cerebrum
pituitary gland
nose
cerebellum
head
neck
thyroid gland
heart
lung, bronchus
plexus
stomach
pancreas
duodenum
ureter
intestine
uterus
hemorrhoid

frontal sinus
eyes
ear, tonsil
trapezius muscle
shoulder
liver
adrenal gland
gall
kidney
transverse colon
ascending colon
caecum
knee and bottom
ovary, testicle

180

Scoliosis pain

You can wand the back with someone with scoliosis but there are other effective places to wand as well. Wanding the top of the head with the circling technique or the cross-hatching technique can relieve some of the pain and may affect the alignment positively.

Place your little finger against the base of your ear with your hand resting on your neck. With your thumb, mark the spot on your neck. Try to align your thumb in a straight line vertically from your ear. Use the rubbing or rolling technique on that spot.

The other place to work with scoliosis is at the base of the neck in the front of your body. If you feel around on the front of the base of your neck you will feel bones. Find the midline of your neck, then move two inches or so either side of your neck. You will feel a sore spot where this place is. Feel around for it. Use the rubbing or rolling technique there.

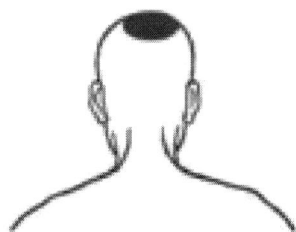

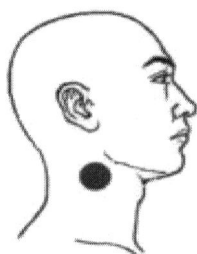

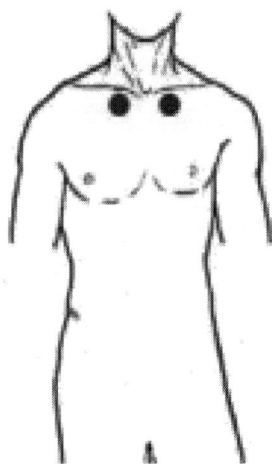

Shoulder Pain

Wanding the shoulder itself is a good start. Depending on how deep the pain is will depend on which technique to use. Deep pain needs the dipping, circle dipping, tip tapping or even either of the cross-hatching techniques. More shallow pain can be wanded with a circular technique.

If you wand the opposite hip to the shoulder that is sore with a dipping or circle dipping technique, you can sometimes get relief.

Believe it or not, a good remedy for shoulder pain is to use the wand on the knuckle of the first finger by using the rolling or rubbing technique.

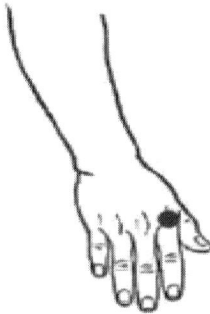

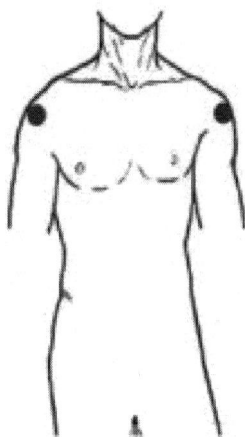

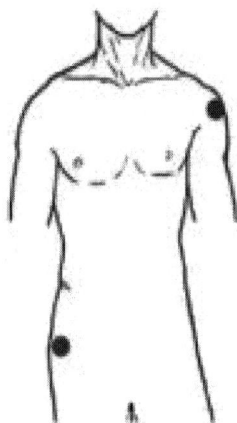

Sprains

Working on location with muscle sprains is best. After you have iced the part and had it checked for breaks, you can begin wanding to repair stretched and torn muscle fibers use the dipping, circle dipping, dotting, tip tapping or any cross-hatching technique so that it penetrates to the depth of the muscles, tendons and ligaments.

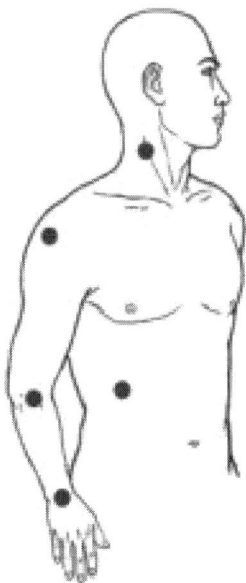

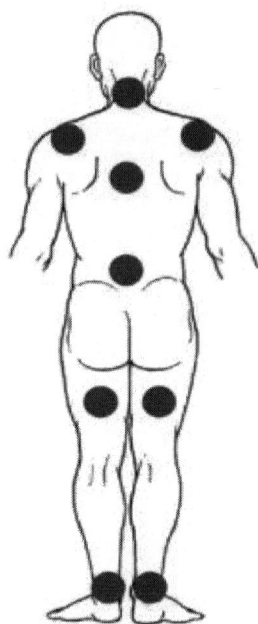

Stomach Problems, Digestive Upsets

One technique that could work very well for stomach problems is to wand in circles around your knees making sure you are wanding upwards on the inside of your knees.

For digestive upsets there is a place on the back of your hand that you can wand which will help cramping and diarrhea. Bend your fingers so you can see your knuckles. One finger width from the knuckle of the first finger, towards the wrist, is a spot that if you use the rolling technique of the rubbing technique may relieve your cramping and diarrhea.

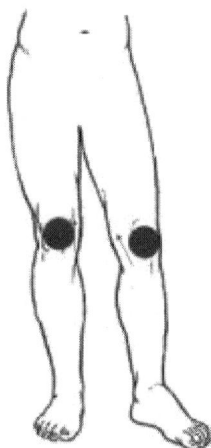

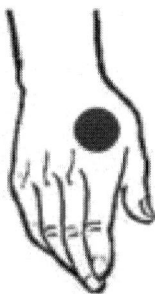

191

Stress

Stress is endemic in society. We decide to do too much, we don't have enough 'me' time, so we get stressed and worn out. The clockwise circular technique is one of the best for stress. Wand the thymus area of the chest in the front, which is one handwidth below the base of the neck.

If you need more energy, there is a place on both legs that you can wand as well. Bend your knee slightly so you can feel where the base of your kneecap is. One handwidth below that is an indent, on the inside of the leg just about two finger widths to the left of the center of your leg on your right leg and two finger widths to the right on your left leg. Use the rolling technique on each leg.

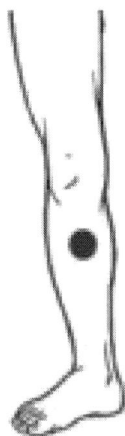

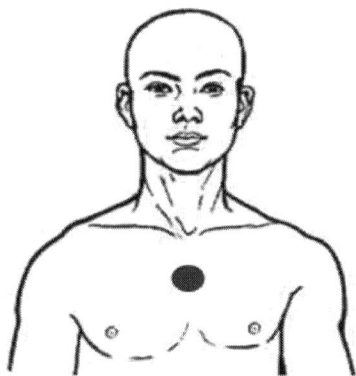

Strokes

To relieve some of the symptoms of strokes there are several places you can use the wand. The first place is in the middle of the bottom of each foot where the ball of the foot meets the arch. Use the rolling, rubbing or dipping technique there.

Another place to relieve symptoms is on the middle of the inside of the wrist about three finger widths up from the wrist crease. Use the circle dipping, dipping, rolling or rubbing technique there.

The next place you can wand is directly under the nose. Wand the center of the septum, where the nose joins the face, using the rolling technique.

Just behind the ear toward the back of the head is a bump that bulges out of the head. Wand that spot with a circular rubbing technique, being sure to wand the whole bump on either side of the head.

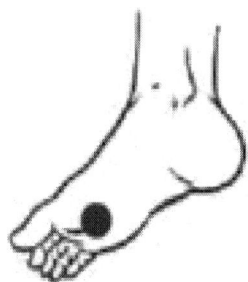

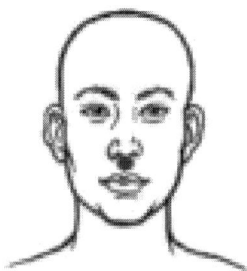

195

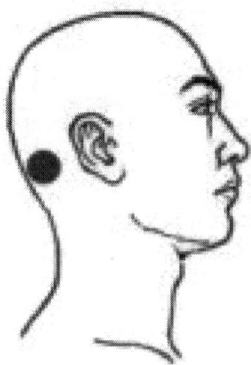

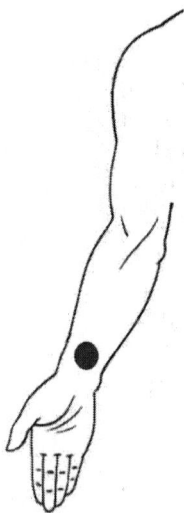

196

Swelling

Swelling is inflammation regardless whether it is from injury or an organic cause. The cross hatching technique or the zigzag cross-hatching technique, followed by the clockwise circling technique is an effective technique.

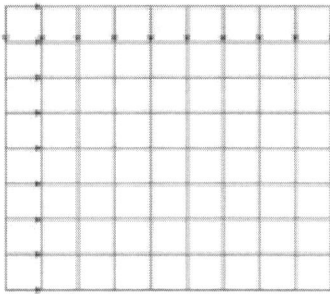

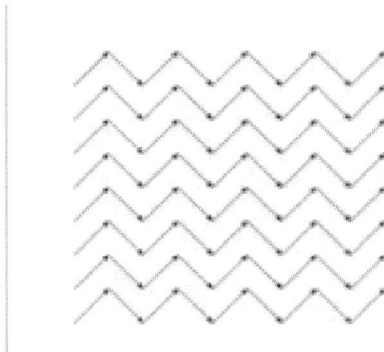

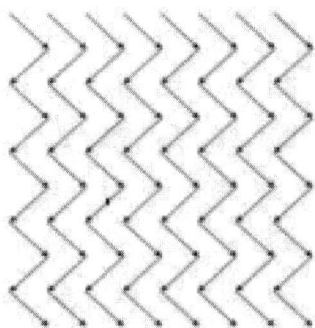

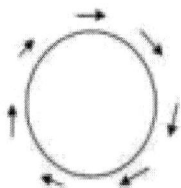

Tinnitus

Tinnitus can be extremely annoying especially if it appears to be loud. The first place to wand is over the ear with a circular or dipping technique.

Another place that is effective is on the back of each hand between the little finger and the ring finger about one half inch in from where the finger webbing is. Rub or roll the wand on that spot.

The next effective place to reduce tinnitus is from the top of each ear, behind to the bottom of the ear. Use the rubbing technique or a stroking technique behind the ear.

You may also reduce your tinnitus by rolling or rubbing your wand at your waistband at the back on either side of your spine.

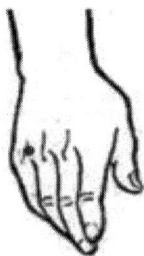
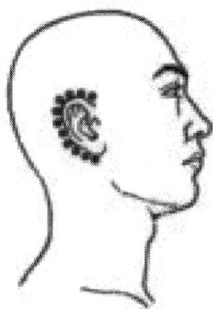

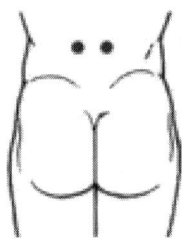

Trigeminal Neuralgia

Western medicine apparently has no cure for this very painful condition. Some people suffer with it for years. Try this technique and see if you get some relief. Turn your hand vertically so that your thumb is on the top, your little finger is on the bottom and your palm is on the side. Lift your thumb so that it is sticking up. Place two fingers against your raised thumb on your wrist. Stick your wand on the spot by your outside finger on top of your arm and use the rubbing or rolling technique there. Do the spot on the other arm.

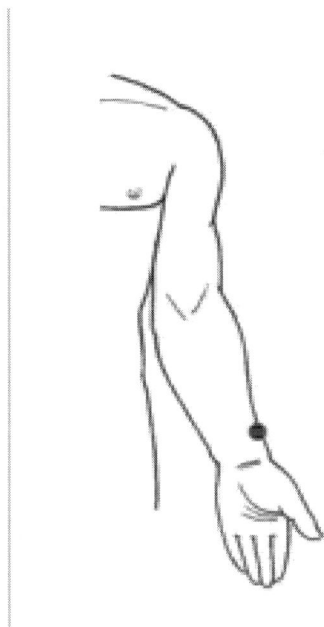

Trigger Points

Trigger points are small groups of tightly contracted muscle fibers within a muscle that are painful or translate pain to a nearby area. They are not as big as a whole muscle spasm, but they hurt nonetheless. The tight contraction cuts off its own microcirculation which intensifies the pain even more. Toxins build up, oxygen is depleted and the area become a toxic swamp. The contracted muscle fibers or knots are called trigger points. This is very familiar in conditions like fibromyalgia. By feeling where the soreness is and finding the sorest spot, roll the wand between your thumb and your first finger at the skin surface or slightly above the skin surface. Only put as much pressure on the skin as is tolerable. Roll the spot until you feel it release. It is important that the wand move. Just holding it on the spot won't quite do the job.

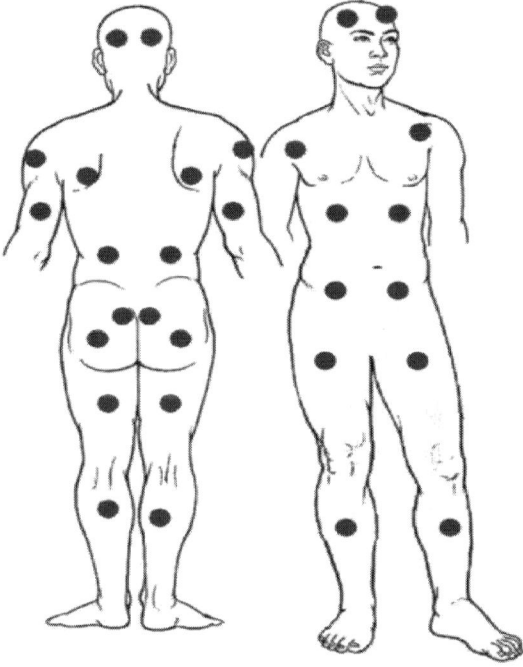

Vertigo

There are a few places on the body that help with dizziness. One is on the inside of the wrist where the arm connects to each hand. There is a groove felt in the middle of the wrist. Use the rubbing or rolling technique there.

Another spot is in the middle of the ball of each foot near the arch. You will feel a groove there where you can use rolling or rubbing technique.

You can also roll or rub your wand on your back, either side of your spine where the waistband of your pants sits.

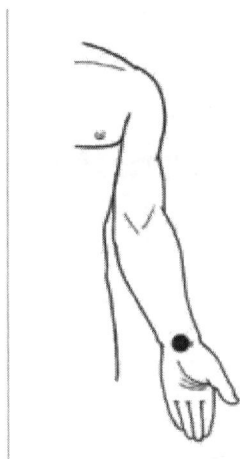

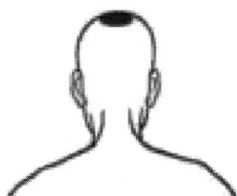

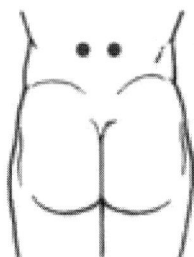

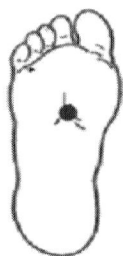

209

Vomiting

The fastest way to control vomiting is to use the rolling technique on the point on the ball of each foot where the groove is felt just above the arch.

You can also wand on the lower outside of the knee with a rolling or rubbing technique.

Another good place to relieve vomiting is on the inside of the wrist, two finger widths above the crease in the wrist. Any of the wanding techniques work but you may want to use the rolling or rubbing technique making skin contact.

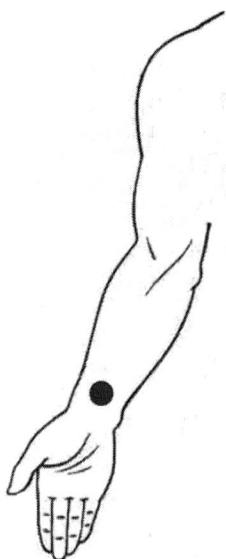

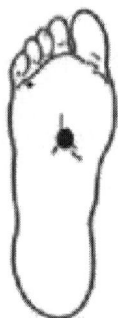

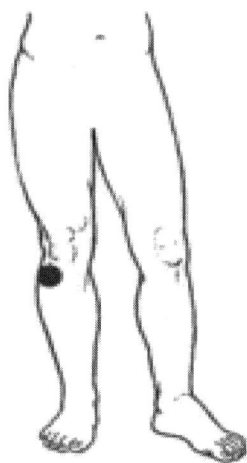

There are many other conditions that can be helped by using a zero-point energy wand and by using the variety of techniques shown early on in the book, you can find the most effective ones for you, your body begins to heal and you have become the healer that you innately are.

Congratulations on realizing you can heal yourself. You have just opened the door to amazing experiences and insights into a whole new world. You will soon be stretching your horizons even further. We encourage you to read and research into alternative ways to improve your health still further. Discuss these with your medical health practitioner and implement them into your life. Pretty soon, you could be a whole new person. We are proud to walk with you on that journey.

Structured Water

What is it?

More important then the chemical make up of water is the structure of water. Water has been found to have memory and it remembers information from the last environment it had contact with. There is a reason why our ancestors used silver as serving containers for food and water.

Dr. Masaru Emoto has done extensive research in this area and many of his videos showing crystals of frozen structured water are available on Youtube.

Books are being written and are showing up Amazon about structured water and trying to explain everything in a short excerpt would not do the subject justice. Be sure to visit Amazon to find books available on this subject.

Here is an important aspect of what structured water can do. When one takes structured water and pours it into a container of water that is not structured, the complete vessel of water becomes structured.

Since we can change a larger amount of water using a smaller amount of structured water, self healers and parishioners should take this into account. Our brains are 94% water and our bodies being mostly water and there are so many negative vibrations in the world that the water in our bodies is constantly being bombarded by these negative waves and frequencies. As individuals, we even affect the structure of the water in our bodies by our very thoughts. People who think about being sick all the time are sick all the time and those who think about being healthy all the time are healthy all the time.

Having a way to restored the water in our bodies to a positive vibration is important for our health and well-being.

When we drink a glass of very cold water and then place our palm over our forehead, we can feel that the temperature of our forehead is colder for a short period. This is because as soon as we drink water, our brain is immediately re-hydrated with the new water.

I heard an expert in this area once explain it this way. He said "in simple terms" that there are a couple of small tubes that go from our stomach to our brains. Once water enters the stomach (not coffer, tea, orange juice or other liquids) it is converted to another chemical which is immediately shot up into our brain. This re-hydrates the brain. The brain is not re-hydrated by the blood system but via this stomach-brain connection.

Since this re-hydration process occurs immediately once we have taken in water, by drinking structured water we can expect that the water in our brains, as well as the water in our bodies, will be affected after we ingest the water. So by drinking structured water we can affect the water in our brain immediately creating a positive affect which can help us toward becoming healthier.

How can you get "structured water"?

While there are companies selling expensive units that can create structured water, Goldwell suggest people with limited means use the oldest technique known to mankind and that is to say a prayer before ingesting water, food and other liquids. It has been found that water that has been blessed has been transformed from being erratic to being structured.

As shown in Dr. Emoto's research, saying something nice and sending good thoughts to the water one is about to drink also affects the water. Once you fill a glass with water you are about to drink, it is best to at the very least say something positive and uplifting to the water.

Since it has been found that water retains the frequencies of thoughts and other vibrations in it's surroundings, Goldwell further suggest to others that they use a 528 hz frequency that has been used by alternative healing practitioners and others and is referred to as the DNA repair frequency.

Last, but not least, Goldwell also suggest that those that own zero point energy wands treat their water with their wand either by waving the wand over the water or by simply placing the wand in the water and letting it stand for a minute or so before drinking.

Goldwell uses what is known as an Iyashi zero point energy wand which has been infused with 1700 healing frequencies. No matter what wand a person uses, treating water with a ZPE wand is more advantageous then not at all.

Bruce Goldwell has created a short video explaining how to make structured water using a zero point energy wand and the 528 hz frequency.

This video is available at:

http://www.youtube.com/watch?v=CGIaDT60_bg

The 528 hz frequency is available at:

http://www.youtube.com/watch?v=26TO9Nk3ENg

To make it easy for people to visit these links online, Goldwell has provided the links on his web site at:

www.BruceGoldwell.com

Much is yet to be discovered about how water can be used for healing the body and we expect in the very near future more evidence will be provided by those who are researching this issue.

In the meantime, we as individuals can start right now to transform our lives and live healthier lifestyles by taking matters into our own hands. Being sure to take advantage of the miracle of structured water is a huge step in the right direction.

AUTHORS

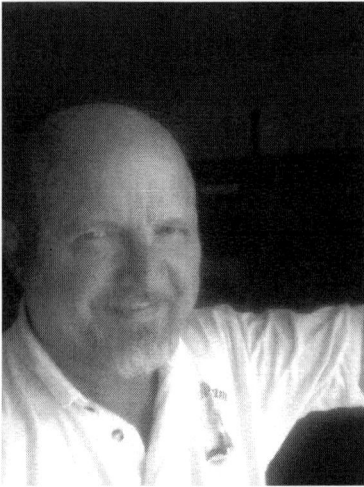

Bruce Goldwell

Bruce has over a dozen books in publication. Not only does he write book about self-help, his is also the author of the "Dragon Keepers" series which is a fantasy adventure for young readers. Bruce has embedded success principles in the "Dragon Keepers" books so that young readers can learn these principles while experiencing the fantasy, mystery and adventure of the Dragon Keepers series.

Bruce is the father of six children and has ten grandchildren. He is currently single and lives on the Treasure Coast in sunny Florida.

Mr. Goldwell is an advocate of alternative healing. One of his missions in life is to help people to experience abundant health, wealth and happiness. He believes that wanding will play a primary role in helping people to achieve optimum health and wellness.

Web site: www.BruceGoldwell.com

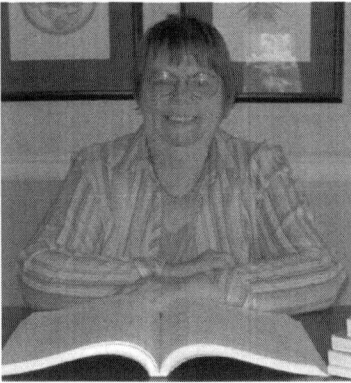

Jean Perrins

Jean Perrins is a medical intuitive, expert energy practitioner and instructor, professional copywriter, article writer, author and health coach. She is an expert platinum writer for Ezinearticles.com and is involved with several other blogs and websites. Her knowledge and expertise in the water ionization and remediation business is well known. She is also involved with two other companies, both of which are green innovative businesses that will make a difference in environmental and personal health.

She lives in a small beach town in British Columbia near the US border with her son, two dogs, two cats and four birds. She enjoys gardening, drawing, cooking, beadwork, biking, going to the gym, walking and working with the plethora of local and distance clients that make her acquaintance. She knows how to squeeze every ounce of health into a body.

Made in the USA
San Bernardino, CA
04 May 2014